Principles of Mechanics and Biomechanics

STOC DYNNWYD YMAITH
LLYFRGELL COLEG MENAI
WITHDRAWN LIBRARY STOCK

D0306758

Principles of Mechanics and Biomechanics

Frank Bell

Glasgow Caledonian University
Glasgow, UK

LLYFRGELL COLEG MENAI LIBRARY
SAFLE FFRIDDOEDD SITE
BANGOR GWYNEDD LL57 2TP

Stanley Thornes (Publishers) Ltd

© 1998 Stanley Thornes (Publishers) Ltd

All rights reserved. No part of this publication may be reproduced or transmitted in any form or by any means, electronic or mechanical, including photocopying, recording or any information storage and retrieval system, without permission in writing from the publisher or under licence from the Copyright Licensing Agency Limited. Further details of such licences (for reprographic reproduction) may be obtained from the Copyright Licensing Agency Limited, of 90 Tottenham Court Road, London W1P 9HE.

First published in 1998 by:
Stanley Thornes (Publishers) Ltd
Ellenborough House
Wellington Street
CHELTENHAM
GL50 1YW
United Kingdom

98 99 00 01 02 / 10 9 8 7 6 5 4 3 2 1

A catalogue record for this book is available from the British Library

ISBN 0-7487-3332-9

ST NO	0748733329
ACC NO	047584
CLASS	612.76
DATE	27.03.01
STAFF	AR

Typeset by Northern Phototypesetting Co. Ltd, Bolton, UK
Printed and bound in Great Britain
by Scotprint Ltd, Musselburgh, Scotland

Dedication

To Cathy, Mark and Craig

Contents

Preface

Biomechanics can provide professionals such as medical engineers, occupational therapists, physiotherapists and sports scientists with a powerful, analytical tool for evaluating many clinical problems. In this book the essential common core of principles of mechanics and biomechanics necessary for a basic understanding of the science are gathered together.

An imaginative approach is required at the start of the study of biomechanics if the relevance to clinical practice is to be established and the intellectual curiosity of the reader stimulated. In clinical practice biomechanical problems do not present themselves in nice, clear cut textbook style. Patients do not move about in one convenient **plane** with **centres of gravity** and **force vectors** pinned to their bodies but clinicians such as physiotherapists still need to appreciate the presence and significance of forces acting on and within the patient's body.

At the beginning of Chapter 1 a case study is introduced based on an elderly patient who had muscle weakness resulting from a circulatory problem. He presented almost classical illustrations of problems amenable to biomechanical analysis when he attempted typical daily acts of living such as rising from a chair, standing on one leg and walking with a walking frame. Reference is made to this case study in three of the first four chapters which cover the essential foundation of **statics**.

Chapter 5 deals with **principles of machines**, a topic which is becoming more important with the increasing use of exercise machines and work simulator devices in rehabilitation.

Structures and materials, **dynamics** and **fluid mechanics** are introduced in Chapters 6, 7 and 8, respectively.

These eight chapters provide the reader with a basic-level text that introduces important concepts in mechanics applied to the human body, remedial equipment, materials, tissues, structures and fluids without reference to controversial issues and requiring very little mathematical skill or knowledge.

Tutorial problems are included at the end of each chapter and should be regarded as an integral part of the text. Answers to tutorial problems can be found at the back of the book. A brief discussion of research-based sources of information is included in the Appendix.

What is biomechanics? | 1

CHAPTER OVERVIEW

This chapter introduces the particular branch of science known as bio-mechanics, indicates the scope of the related disciplines (as listed in the key words, below) and introduces a case study to illustrate the relevance of biomechanics to professionals such as medical engineers, occupational therapists and physiotherapists. The value and the limitations of personal everyday experience in understanding biomechanical phenomena are stressed. Suggestions on how to use this book in a planned study pro-gramme on biomechanics are given.

KEY WORDS

- Mechanics
- Biomechanics
- Dynamics, kinematics, kinetics
- Statics
- Rigid body
- Solid deformable body
- Fluid

1.1 INTRODUCTION: A CASE STUDY

This case study is based on an elderly man who, following rupture of a major blood vessel (the aorta), suffered considerable weakness in the muscles around his abdominal region, his pelvis and his legs (e.g. the hip extensors – the muscles that can extend or 'pull back' the trunk if it is flexed forward over the thighs; and the hip abductors – the muscles surrounding the hip that can pull and straighten the trunk if it is leaning over to the opposite side). The case notes are summarized in more clinical terms in Table 1.1.

This patient presented almost classical illustrations of the types of problem amenable to biomechanical analysis when he attempted typical daily acts of living such as rising from a chair, standing on one leg and walking with a walking frame (Figure 1.1).

We will apply the material presented in Chapters 2 and 3 to examine different aspects of this case. At this stage it would be useful for the reader to observe and practise two of the above tasks.

- Try rising from a chair without using your arms to assist; note the sequence of actions involved and the position of your feet and trunk. The patient under consideration has weak hip extensors (see brief description above); what effect would this have?
- Standing erect, put your right hand over your right hip; now take your left foot off the floor; can you feel the muscles over your right hip tense when you do this? This is your hip abductors contracting. The above patient has weak hip abductors; what effect would this have?

Table 1.1   Case study clinical notes

An 80-year-old retired teacher who had an aortic aneurysm that necessitated Y-graft surgery. Postoperatively he was hypotensive, in acute renal failure and suffered cord ischaemia. This latter resulted in gross weakness of his gluteal muscles and his abdominal muscles.
His muscle strength when assessed was:

Right hip extensors	Grade 2
Left hip extensors	Grade 3
Right hip abductors	Grade 2+
Left hip abductors	Grade 2
Right hamstrings (as knee flexors)	Grade 2
Left hamstrings (as knee flexors)	Grade 3

(The above was based on the six-point Oxford scale, in which strength is assessed from 0 = no contraction to 5 = normal.)
His rehabilitation had reached the point where he was mobile on a walking frame and was managing to ascend and descend stairs.

1.2   MECHANICS AND BIOMECHANICS

The word 'biomechanics' is made up of two roots; *bio*, meaning life (Greek, *bios*, way of life), and *mechanics*.

1.2.1   Mechanics

Mechanics is a branch of science that deals with forces and the effects of forces, specifically the motion and deformation of solid, liquid and gaseous matter.

Although this branch of science is based on relatively few basic laws the range of application and the characteristic methods of applying these basic laws are so extensive that across this branch there are a number of subjects that are themselves regarded as definite disciplines. Three of these disciplines are: the **mechanics of rigid bodies** (itself comprising statics, kinematics and kinetics), the **mechanics of solid deformable bodies** (solid materials and structures) and **fluid mechanics** (liquids and gases). Each of these three disciplines can be applied usefully in the theory and practice of remedial therapy in understanding the principles of the use of therapy apparatus, human movement, injury and the prevention and treatment of physical disorders.

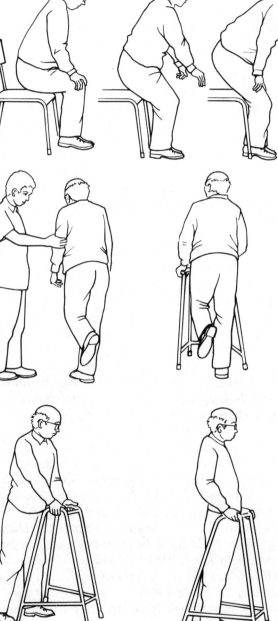
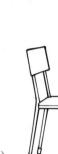
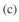

Figure 1.1 Case study: patient with muscle weakness. (**a**) Attempting to rise from a chair. (**b**) Attempting to stand on one leg. (**c**) Walking with the aid of a walking frame.

Every adult has a wide range of experience of the main phenomena in mechanics – force, motion and deformation. Throughout our lives we experience muscular forces in the form of pushes and pulls, the movements that can result from such forces and, sometimes, the painful and destructive deformations and mechanical failures that force can cause. The cornerstone of mechanics is also based on experiences; Newton's three basic laws of motion are essentially statements of experience that could not be derived from logic or mathematical analysis alone. In arriving at these laws, however, the 'experience' of scientists such as Galileo and Newton included that based on careful observation, measurement and experimentation.

The foundation on which classical mechanics rests involves the concepts of mass, length, time, force, Newton's laws of motion and the rules of geometry, arithmetic, algebra, trigonometry and calculus. The three disciplines of mechanics that are introduced in this book are based on this foundation but each involves, in addition, its own characteristic concepts, principles, techniques and specialized data found from experimentation.

1.2.2 Words of caution and encouragement

It will be apparent, even at this very early point in the text, that to gain some proficiency in understanding and applying the principles of mechanics it is necessary to learn a new vocabulary and that familiarity with this vocabulary requires learning definitions of terms. This is unavoidable but it is also a feature of most disciplines relevant to therapists; anatomy is a particularly good example of such a discipline. Few people are prepared to make the effort unless they can see the relevance and value of the end result. Add to this potential problem of vocabulary the spectre of mathematics and the subject becomes decidedly unattractive to health professionals. Only basic arithmetic, the simplest equations in algebra and graphical methods (as an alternative to trigonometry) are used in this book. Motivation based only on the need to pass a course or an examination reflects poorly on either the perceived relevance of the course or the standard of presentation of the material. Learning involves association: associating a new idea with some familiar ideas or experiences. The closer the associations the clearer the insight and the sense of understanding. This is one very good reason why students should refer to more than one book or source of reference material in any subject, to find associations or examples with which they feel familiar. Associating the concept of force with muscular pushes and pulls is a particularly fortuitous association for therapists. Understanding other manifestations of force can be more difficult. The idea of the force of gravity can be conceived by a combination of acceptance of the idea of muscular force and our everyday experience of weight, even though, in the latter case, the transmission of force seems less visible than that of the push or pull of a limb.

Why does an ice skater spin faster when she draws her outstretched arms inwards towards the side of her body? The conventional answer is often 'because of the conservation of angular momentum'. Momentum is to do with a combination of body mass and motion (momentum is mass × velocity), angular momentum refers to a body mass undergoing circular motion, and conservation of momentum is one of the 'principles' used in analysing certain types of mechanical problem; these concepts are discussed in Chapter 7. At this stage I simply want to pose the question 'does the phenomenon really occur **because** of momentum?' or would it be more reasonable to say that the phenomenon occurs and the principle of the conservation of momentum can be used to predict and describe this and many other similar phenomena? If you have little personal experience of similar 'rotating' phenomena then grasping this principle by association can be problematic. The concept of angular motion is very relevant to the therapist because motion of the human body occurs primarily by angular movement of limbs around joints; for example we walk in a straight line by swinging our thighs, legs and feet through a series of arcs.

It is also important to be aware of the limitations of our own observations and our intuition. The strength of science lies in the fact that statements made are repeatedly tested by measurement by different observers before they are accepted.

Why do objects fall to the ground? Because of gravity! We have already explored the possible limitations of this type of question and answer in relation to the spinning skater. Perhaps in the case of falling objects there is no real problem in understanding because our own observation and experience of this phenomenon is wider than our experience of rotating bodies? Would a heavy adult fall faster than a light child if they both stepped off a diving board at the same time? The answer is no. Both would fall at the same rate and both would strike the water at the same time. The relationships between force (of which weight is an example) and motion are **not** obvious. It took nearly 2000 years for the misconceptions that were taught by the Greeks to be challenged and another 500 years to develop the science of mechanics to its present precise state. Personal experience and intuition have to be supported or refuted by measurement and experimentation.

The subject of mechanics is challenging but it is important that professionals such as therapists and engineers share enough common knowledge of the basic principles and language to ensure its effective application to appropriate healthcare problems.

1.2.3 Biomechanics

The term biomechanics is a very useful label. For example an article entitled 'The mechanics of human movement' could well be concerned with the logistics of installing escalators in public buildings or the problems of controlling an urban transit system or a social study of emigration and immigration. 'The biomechanics of human movement' is more likely to be concerned with some aspect of the human musculoskeletal system. Similarly, one might expect an article entitled 'The biomechanics of a rehabilitation electronic cycle' to be concerned with the forces that act on the patient who uses the equipment and not the forces on the components that comprise the equipment.

If the term is to be defined then we need only modify that used for mechanics to include some appropriate reference to the root, *bio* (life), such as the following. 'Biomechanics is a branch of science that deals with forces and the effects of forces on living systems and matter', i.e. for our purposes it is the application of mechanics to the human body.

1.3 THE USE OF STATICS

During the common activities of daily living the forces transmitted through the joints, limbs and tissues of the body can be well in excess of the body weight of the individual. When rising from a chair, forces on the knee joints can reach values some three or four times the value of body weight, and in particularly unfavourable conditions, even higher. Those responsible for designing or selecting furniture and equipment for the elderly and disabled should be aware of this as should those health professionals who treat and advise the elderly and disabled.

Bending over to lift an object (or a patient) can generate forces in the lumbar region of the back as high as ten times the load being lifted if the technique used is poor. Understanding how the magnitude of the stress imposed on the back is related to the geometry of the lifter is an important step in understanding and preventing lower back pain and injury, a problem which, it is worth noting, is as prevalent in healthcare workers as it is in many other less well informed groups of workers.

When simply walking at a relatively normal speed, the forces transmitted through the joints of the lower limbs can rise and fall between two and five times body weight. Indeed, the force across the hip joint may be two to three times body weight when one is just standing still on one leg (Figures 1.2 (e, f)). Perhaps even more surprising, though, is the suggestion that a patient, lying in bed, may generate forces in the hip in excess of body weight by attempting to raise a leg clear of the bed. Before a therapist selects a **non-weightbearing** exercise or activity, for a patient to avoid premature stressing of an injured limb or joint, it is worth while reflecting on the fact that the forces acting within the body may be much higher than one intuitively expects. This magnification of forces within the body is not something that is obvious but the mechanism can be better understood by the concepts of levers (and moments of force), which are dealt with in that part of mechanics called **statics**.

In statics, the body (this term can refer to an inanimate object as well as the human body or parts of the body) is viewed as stationary, i.e. at rest, and certain rules that must govern forces acting on a body at rest are applied. This involves the concept of levers. It is a powerful and valuable concept that can be applied to many practical problems in remedial therapy. When an occupational therapist suggests that an elderly or disabled client uses a long-handled tap rather than a conventional one this is to provide good leverage (Figures 1.2 (a, b)). Similarly when the physiotherapist applies manual resistance or assistance to the movement of a patient's limb, by applying force at the end of the limb, the force required from the therapist is reduced as leverage is increased (Figures 1.2 (c, d)). When standing on one leg, the force on the supporting hip joint may exceed the apparent weight acting on the joint because of the effect of internal leverage (Figures 1.2 (e, f)). A patient with a painful hip may lean over to the affected hip, contrary to our intuition, in an attempt to eliminate this leverage effect (Figures 1.2 (g, h)).

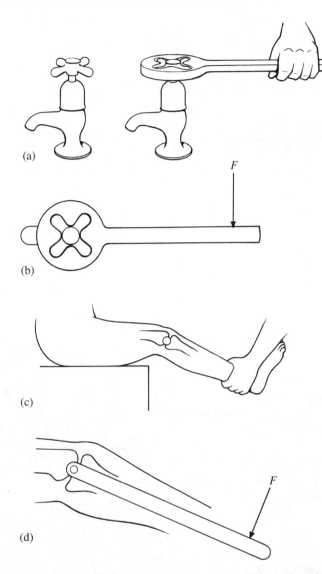

Figure 1.2 The concept of levers. (**a, b**) Leverage provided by a long-handled tap. (**c, d**) Leverage about the knee joint. (**e, f**) Leverage of body weight about the hip joint during unilateral stance. (**g, h**) Eliminating leverage about the hip joint by leaning over the joint.

   Although it has been stated above that in statics the body is viewed as stationary, fortunately the methods of statics can be applied to moving bodies provided that certain basic rules are followed. In essence we analyse the moving body at instants in time when we can define and measure the geometry of the body; in effect we analyse snapshots of the moving body to examine the external and internal forces that must be acting. In fact, examining the motion of a body *per se* even without reference to forces can itself provide valuable information for the therapist; this is the topic of **kinematics**.

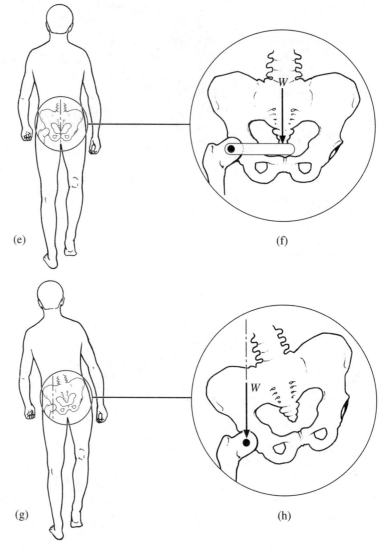

Figure 1.2 continued

1.4 THE USE OF KINEMATICS

Kinematics can be described as the geometry of motion. Maintaining the potential for motion or movement in patients who are otherwise 'immobilized' and restoring optimum capability for motion in patients is a major goal in many rehabilitation programmes. Judgements on what constitutes normal and abnormal motion require some form of statement from the observer. Kinematics provides a quantification and precision to these statements. For example, in examining pathological walking patterns or the 'gaits' of patients, while it is still useful to identify characteristic 'limps', it is proving more useful to use the systematic methods developed in kinematics. Parameters such as length, displacement, angle and time can be estimated or measured and recorded. Observations are made on each body segment or joint (trunk, pelvis, hip, knee, ankle and foot) in addition to the body as a whole. This approach not only contributes to rationalizing the diagnosis of the origin of locomotor problems but also makes the comparison of treatment regimes and the recording of the progress of patients more universal and reliable than that based solely on the subjective and personal experience of skilled clinicians. The area of gait analysis is a good example of the type of activity where collaboration between medical engineers and clinicians, such as orthopaedic consultants or physiotherapists, can be very fruitful.

The use of kinematics is not limited to gait analysis. The analysis of motion is the first step in examining another type of force which is relevant to the therapist – dynamic forces. Dynamic forces are dealt with in the branch of mechanics called **kinetics**.

1.5   THE USE OF KINETICS

Which of the following incidents would cause most pain and injury: gently placing a 1 kg block of cast iron on to your foot or dropping the block on to your foot from a height of, say, 1 m? Hopefully few people would dispute that the latter case would be the more painful and destructive.

Forces are required to start motion, to change motion and, as in the case of the falling block of cast iron, to stop motion. The size of the force is directly related to both the mass of the object and the changes that occur in its motion. In gently placing the 1 kg mass on the foot there is little motion involved and consequently little change in motion required; the force on the foot in this case is just the weight of the block. The dropped block, although it is the same mass, will have achieved a reasonable speed before striking the foot; the dynamic force required to stop it moving may be several times the weight of the block. The more rapidly the block is stopped, i.e. the smaller the time interval, the greater the dynamic force.

If the tissues and structures of the foot assist in spreading out the time taken to stop the object then the dynamic forces involved will be reduced; this is known as the shock absorber effect. If the mechanical properties of the material comprising the block are changed again the dynamic forces will be altered. A 1 kg sandbag will produce different dynamic effects from a 1 kg block of cast iron. However, before looking at the mechanical properties of matter we will consider one other general application of kinetics.

Just as a force is required to stop motion, one is also required to start motion. A patient with weak muscles may have difficulty in initiating the movement of a limb but given appropriate assistance to overcome the inertia of the limb the patient may have little difficulty in completing the motion. Equally of course, a patient may consciously or subconsciously use kinetic forces to 'cheat' during exercise regimes, achieving the desired range of motion of a joint by a kicking action of the limb. Hospital and community-based healthcare workers may also use a knowledge of kinetics to considerable effect to minimize the forces required to lift and transfer patients. The applications of the principles of rate of change of motion, momentum and energy, the topics of kinetics, are of practical use.

Appreciating how matter responds to force is also of practical use. The topics of structures, materials and human tissues, and the mechanics of fluids are introduced in Chapters 6 and 8, respectively, but as one aim of the book is to show the integration of these disciplines an indication of their uses in health-care is appropriate here.

1.6   RIGID AND NON-RIGID BODIES

A rigid body is one whose size and shape are not affected by the forces acting on it. It is one of a number of useful theoretical concepts that allow us to begin to examine real problems without the added complications of also dealing with the changing geometry of the body, for example. Real solid bodies of course are not rigid, they deform under load. The internal effects of forces on a solid structure depend on the characteristics of the external forces, the inherent mechanical properties of the material, such as its strength and stiffness, and the size and shape of the structure. The definitions, principles and laws of the mechanics of solid deformable bodies are being applied in the design and manufacture of medical devices and in the analysis of the human musculoskeletal system to prevent, correct or treat deformities and movement dysfunctions. While most clinicians will not be involved directly in the design of medical devices or in the more complex analyses of the mechanics of human tissues, they do require a basic understanding of such a relevant discipline.

Most solids offer considerable resistance to any force that tends to change their shape. In contrast liquids and gases offer little if any resistance to forces which tend to change their shape, they flow and, hence, the common term **fluid**. The term fluid, therefore, includes both liquids and gases and a number of mechanical principles can be applied to both states of matter although each state of matter also possesses particular characteristics. For the clinician, fluid mechanics is relevant in understanding: blood flow and the influence of posture on blood pressure; the mechanism of breathing and the mechanics of postural drainage; the mechanisms of human joint lubrication; the behaviour of human connective tissues; the use of hydrotherapy in patient treatment; and the properties of some specific aids and equipment for the disabled that make use of pneumatic or hydraulic principles.

1.7   NOTES FOR STUDENTS

1.7.1   Summaries and revision

Summaries of individual chapters are provided in the book; however, as preparing succinct notes on lectures, seminars and reading material is one of the skills that students must develop to improve their own learning strategies, they are advised to attempt to produce their own summary notes before looking at these. The chapter overviews and key words at the front of each chapter can be used to plan summary and revision notes.

1.7.2 Definitions of terms

In science, definitions are used to express concisely and unequivocally the facts and concepts. Unfortunately, in examinations students are often requested to 'define' certain terms or basic laws, but few students after one year of study can really be expected to have a 'concise and unequivocal' understanding of a subject, and hence most tend to memorize definitions without necessarily understanding the nuances of the words used. Precision in language is one of the hallmarks of science, but it can be developed. The first requirement for students is to develop an interest in the subject and to build up associations of ideas that give them confidence in their understanding and eventual application of knowledge of the subject.

1.7.3 Tutorials

Tutorial problems are given at the end of each chapter and answers are given at the end of the book. They are generally limited to what would be expected to be reasonably tackled in a 1 hour tutorial session and should be treated as an integral part of the text.

1.7.4 Holistic care and integrated studies

Professional staff are expected to be able to draw on all of their knowledge and practical skills in the safe evaluation and treatment of patients; the term **holistic care** implies seeing the needs and problems of the whole patient. The principles of biomechanics can be applied to a wide range of phenomena but movement and movement dysfunction, injury, disorder and treatment are not subject only to mechanical principles. It is important that students themselves attempt to relate 'subjects' of study whenever possible and that they question and challenge the role of any particular piece of knowledge to their professional needs; students and teachers both benefit from this questioning attitude.

1.8   SUMMARY

Mechanics is a branch of science that deals with **forces** and the effects of forces, specifically the **motion** and **deformation** of matter.
Biomechanics is the application of mechanics to the human body.
    Three important disciplines within mechanics are:
- the **mechanics of rigid bodies** (statics, kinematics and kinetics);
- the mechanics of **solid deformable bodies** (solid materials and structures); and
- **fluid mechanics** (liquids and gases).

During activities of daily living, forces transmitted through the joints, limbs and tissues of the body can be many times the body weight of the individual; the concept of **leverage** (**moments of force**) explains this phenomenon.

1.9 TUTORIAL PROBLEMS

1. A number of terms have been used in this chapter without definition or example of the meaning. While most of these terms are used in everyday language, in science they have precise meanings. The scientific meaning of these terms are developed in subsequent chapters where it is more appropriate. Make a list of all of the terms that are new to you.
2. A patient weighing 500 newtons (N) stands on one leg.
   (a) What size of force is likely to be acting across the supporting hip joint?
   (b) What concept in mechanics helps to explain the size of this force in relation to the patient's body weight?
   (c) What action can the patient take to reduce the size of this force?
3. (a) What is meant by the term kinematics?
   (b) Give one practical example where kinematics can be used in patient assessment.
4. What is meant by a 'dynamic force'?

(See Answers section at the end of this book.)

Is it moving? Force and moment of force

2

CHAPTER OVERVIEW

It is conventional to begin the study of mechanics with detailed descriptions of the motion of particles and bodies because definitions of concepts such as force and mass require showing the relationships between force and motion as described in Newton's laws of motion. In this chapter the relationship between force and motion is briefly discussed to allow adequate definitions of force, mass and weight to be presented but a detailed description of motion is given in Chapter 7. The main aim of this chapter is to introduce the two essential concepts required for static analysis of biomechanical problems, **force** and **moment of force**.

KEY WORDS

- Mass
- Acceleration
- Inertia
- Gravity
- Weight
- Magnitude

- Vector
- Action force
- Reaction force
- Centre of mass
- Moment of force

2.1 FORCES AND MOTION

The description and analysis of motion is the subject of **kinematics** (*kinema* meaning 'cinema' as in motion pictures). The description and analysis of forces that result in motion is the subject of **kinetics**. The description and analysis of forces that **tend** to cause motion is the subject of **statics**. The qualifying statement 'tend to cause motion' is of major importance in the study of statics. Kinematics and kinetics will be reviewed in some detail in Chapter 7, but many very relevant clinical problems can be examined in terms of statics alone.

In statics we deal primarily with stationary bodies (or objects) although the essential requirement is not that the body is at rest but that if it is moving then its speed is not changing either in magnitude or in direction.

If a single force, such as a push, acts on a body, the body will start to move in the same direction as the force and the speed with which it moves will increase proportionally to the magnitude of the force and the length of time the force acts. If a body does not move in this way when pushed or pulled then there is **more** than one force acting and each force is **tending** to produce contradictory motions that, in effect, are cancelling each other out.

If the single force applied to a body in the form of a push or pull is in line with what is called the **centre of mass** of the body, then every part of the body will move in unison at the same speed in the direction of the push. If it is not in line with this centre then the body will still move in the direction of the push but it will rotate (i.e. turn) as well (Figure 2.1).

To apply statics it is necessary to have some appreciation of the motion that would occur under the action of any force even if, at this stage, it is not necessary to examine in detail the motion that does occur when one or more unopposed forces act.

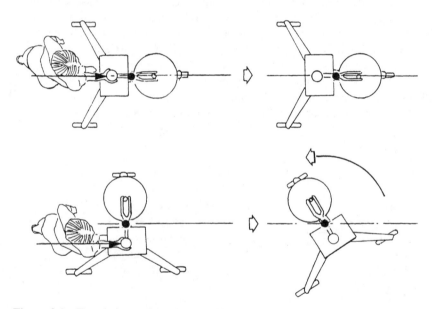

Figure 2.1 Translation and rotation (the black dot represents the centre of gravity).

2.2 INERTIA: NEWTON'S FIRST LAW OF MOTION

The first important relationship between force and motion is given in Newton's first law of motion, which may be stated in the following form:

A body which is at rest will remain at rest unless some external force is applied to it and a body which is moving at a constant speed in a straight line will continue to do so unless some external force is applied to it.

The first part of this statement certainly reflects common experience; stationary objects have to be pushed or pulled to move them. The second part of the statement is not really within common experience. For example, with reference to Figure 2.2, if a patient, using a long handled pusher, pushes a large counter across a board in a therapeutic game of noughts and crosses, usually the counter will come to rest when the person stops pushing. If the surfaces of the counter and board were highly polished then the counter would continue to move for some distance after the person stopped pushing. It can be concluded that in the first case the counter stops almost immediately when the force is removed because there is an opposite force acting due, primarily, to friction between the moving surfaces. When friction is reduced, by polishing the counter and board surfaces, the frictional force opposing motion is reduced; consequently the counter does continue to move for some distance without the need for an external push. Newton's statement, however, implied more than this. If there was **no** resistance whatsoever in the form of surface friction or air resistance (and if the counter board was infinitely long) the counter would continue to move **forever** in a straight line at the speed it had attained at the instant that the push was removed.

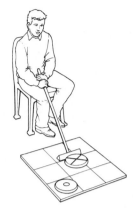

Figure 2.2 Force and motion.

Before considering the next important relationship between force and motion, which is contained in Newton's second law of motion, it would be appropriate to define some of the terms that have now been used.

2.3 DEFINITIONS OF KEY TERMS

Kinematics is the branch of mechanics that is concerned with the phenomenon of motion without reference to mass or force. It may be described as the geometry of motion.

Kinetics is the branch of mechanics that is concerned with motion, mass and the forces that produce motion.

Statics is the branch of mechanics that is concerned with the description and analysis of forces that **tend** to cause motion.

Body is a term used in mechanics to represent any object, animate or inanimate. The term **rigid body** is a theoretical concept used to represent a body whose shape and size are not influenced by external forces.

Magnitude means size and is specified by a number and a unit, e.g. 15 metres, 20 seconds.

Force is a push or a pull. It may be defined by restating Newton's first law of motion:

A force is that which changes or tends to change
the state of rest or uniform motion of a body.

2.4 ACCELERATION: NEWTON'S SECOND LAW OF MOTION

The relationship between force, the resulting motion of a body, and the properties of the body itself, i.e. its size, composition and resistance to motion, are stated in Newton's second law of motion:

$$\text{Force} = \text{mass} \times \text{acceleration}$$
$$\text{i.e. } F = m \times a$$

The italic, m, is used to distinguish mass from the unit of length used in the International System of Units (SI system), which is the metre (m). In this system of units the mass of any body is defined by comparing specific physical behaviours of the body to a 'standard' body. The original standard body in this case is a cylinder of platinum–iridium known as the International Prototype Kilogram, which is stored at the International Bureau of Weights and Measures near Paris. In SI units, the unit of mass is the kilogram (kg).

The properties of the original 'standard' body are its size, composition and its resistance to motion, which in turn is called its **inertia**. Mass may therefore be described as a measure of the quantity of matter in a body (i.e. the quantity of atoms and molecules, where matter is anything that occupies space) and the quantity of inertia possessed by the body. Weight is related to mass but the form of the relationship is sufficiently important to be considered separately.

Acceleration (a) is the rate of change of speed. As speed is measured in metres per second (i.e. m s^{-1}), the rate of change of speed is measured in metres per second per second (i.e. m s^{-2}). If the speed of a body **decreases** this is referred to as **deceleration** but the symbol, a, is still used in this case and the equation $F = m \times a$ is, still applied. What this equation implies is that if the mass of a body is doubled then the force that has to be applied to achieve the same rate of increase of speed, i.e. the same acceleration, must also be doubled. If the force is not doubled the body will still move but at only half the value of acceleration of the first body which had half the mass. The resistance to motion and to change of motion is a property of the body, called **inertia**, related to its mass, and this is a quite separate form of resistance to that caused by other external factors such as friction.

For example, assume that two curling stones have been prepared from the same block of material and that one stone has twice the mass of the other (if the material was absolutely homogeneous, i.e. if its internal composition and structure was uniform throughout then the volume of one stone would be twice that of the other). The two stones are now pushed on a perfectly frictionless ice rink by the same individual using his right hand to push the smaller stone of mass, say, 1 kg, and his left hand to push the larger stone of double the mass, i.e. 2 kg. If he could judge the strength of push of both hands accurately and applied exactly the same force to both stones simultaneously the smaller stone would very quickly move ahead of the larger stone (Figure 2.3). Throughout the short interval that the pushes were being applied, both stones would accelerate but the smaller stone would accelerate twice as much as the larger stone. When he stops pushing, the stones will stop accelerating but both stones will still continue to move in a straight line at the speed that each had attained just before the forces were removed. In this particular case the smaller stone would continue to move at twice the speed of the larger stone (Figure 2.3) and would only slow down or come to rest if some external force, such as friction, acted in the direction opposite to the motion.

To repeat this procedure in such a way that both stones move in perfect unison, i.e. with the same acceleration when the pushes are applied and with identical constant speeds when the pushes are simultaneously removed, the push applied to the large stone would have to be **twice** as great as that applied to the small stone (Figure 2.4).

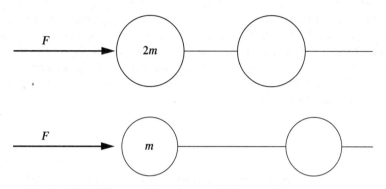

Figure 2.3 Pushing different curling stones with the same force.

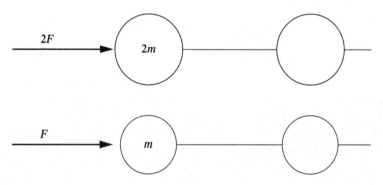

Figure 2.4 Pushing different curling stones with different forces.

The unit of force given in the equation $F = m \times a$ is kg m s^{-2}. For convenience this derived unit is called the newton (N),

i.e. $1 \text{ N} = 1 \text{ kg m s}^{-2}$

2.5 MASS AND WEIGHT

If the two 'curling stones' used in the previous discussion are dropped at the same instant from the same height above the ground, despite the difference in their mass, they would fall in unison with exactly the same acceleration (Figure 2.5).

In fact **all** bodies regardless of mass will fall with the same value of acceleration providing that air resistance is zero or constant. This acceleration of bodies is due to the gravitational pull of the earth. The value of the acceleration due to gravity varies with the distance of the body from the centre of the

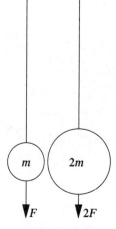

Figure 2.5 Dropping different curling stones.

earth, but the variations in the value of acceleration are very small over the surface of the earth. This acceleration due to gravity is represented by the symbol g, and the value near the surface of the earth in SI units has been found to be 9.8 m s^{-2}.

With respect to the two curling stones, as they are falling vertically in unison this is similar to the case when they were pushed in unison on a horizontal surface; the 2 kg stone required a push twice as great as the 1 kg stone. Similarly when falling in unison the 2 kg stone is being pulled by gravity with a force twice as great as that pulling the 1 kg stone. The pull of gravity is of course called **weight**, thus weight is a force and its value for any body can be calculated from Newton's second law:

Force = mass × acceleration
and weight = mass × acceleration due to gravity
i.e. $W = m \times g$

Example: What is the weight of a body if its mass is one kilogram?

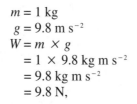

$m = 1$ kg
$g = 9.8$ m s^{-2}
$W = m \times g$
$= 1 \times 9.8$ kg m s^{-2}
$= 9.8$ kg m s^{-2}
$= 9.8$ N,

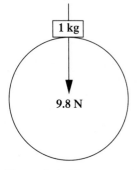

Figure 2.6 Force exerted by the earth on a 1 kg mass.

i.e. the weight of each kilogram mass on the surface of the earth is 9.8 newtons (Figure 2.6; or approximately 10 N). For those who recall the story of Sir Isaac Newton apparently 'discovering gravity' when observing a falling apple, it is appropriate to point out that a medium-sized apple (mass 0.1 kg) has a weight of about 1 N.

2.6   ACTION AND REACTION: NEWTON'S THIRD LAW OF MOTION

When a therapist or a patient pushes or pulls on an object, the object pushes or pulls back. In human locomotion, to move our bodies forward we push backwards on the surface of the ground (Figure 2.7). This fundamental principle is expressed in Newton's third law of motion, which may be stated in the following form:

To every action force there is always opposed an equal reaction force; or the mutual action forces of two bodies upon each other are always equal and oppositely directed.

If human locomotion occurs because the earth, through the medium of surface friction, pushes **us** in the desired direction of motion then surely our push on the earth must in turn move the earth in the opposite direction? In theory it should but the mass of the earth is some hundred thousand, million, million, million times greater than our mass and its acceleration due to our push is consequently that many times less than ours (from Newton's second law, $a = F/m$). In all the problems relevant to therapists this action–reaction principle will involve different bodies that are in contact either directly or through some other matter such as water, but the principle is not restricted to bodies in physical contact. For example, a nail will apply an equal and opposite force on a magnet to that which the magnet applies on the nail even although the bodies are not in contact.

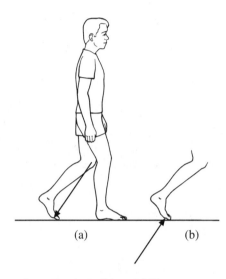

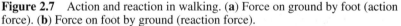

Figure 2.7   Action and reaction in walking. (**a**) Force on ground by foot (action force). (**b**) Force on foot by ground (reaction force).

This pull of both bodies would be sensed if the magnet was held in one hand and the nail in the other hand. Similarly, a falling stone is being pulled to the earth by the gravitational force called its weight but the stone in turn is pulling on the earth (applying a pulling force on the centre of the earth equal to the weight of the stone).

To test a patient's strength a therapist pushes against a patient's limb knowing that the patient must push back with an equal and opposite force. The patient's strength of push may be judged by the therapist in terms of the therapist's strength of push in the opposite direction. The principle of action and reaction is applied at the point of contact of the therapist's hand and the patient's body, i.e. equal and opposite forces act at this common point of contact, but care must be taken in interpreting this force in terms of the internal forces acting within the two bodies (Figure 2.8(a)). Because of the possible difference in internal **leverages** within the patient's body and within the therapist's body, the muscle and joint reaction forces in each case may be **quite different** (Figure 2.8(b)).

The rotation of bodies and the tendency for bodies to rotate because of leverage is dependent on the **moment of force**. Before stating the principle of moment of force the features of the foregoing discussion that are particularly relevant to statics will be briefly listed.

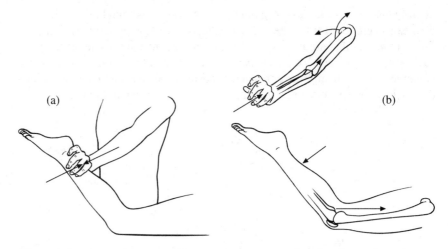

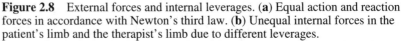

Figure 2.8 External forces and internal leverages. (**a**) Equal action and reaction forces in accordance with Newton's third law. (**b**) Unequal internal forces in the patient's limb and the therapist's limb due to different leverages.

2.7 STATICS: REVIEW OF TERMS

1. In SI units:
   Mass is measured in kilograms (kg)
   Length in metres (m)
   Time in seconds (s)
   Force in newtons (N)
   Care is required when the same letter is used to represent two different words, but this is difficult to avoid. The word mass (m) and the word metre (m) are differentiated by the use of italics.
2. **Mass** is a measure of the quantity of matter that a body contains and the quantity of inertia possessed by the body that resists motion, specifically acceleration. It is a property of a body that does not vary with the location of the body in the universe.
3. **Weight** is a force which, at or near the surface of the earth, is related to the mass of a body by the value of the acceleration due to the gravitational pull of the earth, g, where $g = 9.8$ m s^{-2}. Weight (N) = mass (kg) $\times$ 9.8 m s^{-2}. In other words, the earth exerts a force of 9.8 N on each kg of mass on its surface (Figure 2.6).
   N.B. In tutorial problems a value of $g = 10$ m s^{-2} is a suitable approximation that simplifies computation.

4. A body remains at rest or in uniform motion (i.e. motion at a constant speed in a straight line) unless it is acted upon by an unbalanced set of forces (Newton's first law of motion).
5. To every action force there is an equal and opposite reaction force (Newton's third law of motion). The action force and the reaction force act on different bodies.
6. **Characteristics of a force:** To fully describe a force, four characteristics must be known (e.g. with reference to Figure 2.9)
   (a) its magnitude (e.g. 40 N),
   (b) its line of action (e.g. vertical),
   (c) its direction or sense (e.g. downwards),
   (d) its point of application.
7. Force is a **vector** quantity, i.e. both magnitude and direction must be specified to describe a force. A vector quantity can be represented by a directed straight line drawn to scale, e.g. as in Figure 2.9.

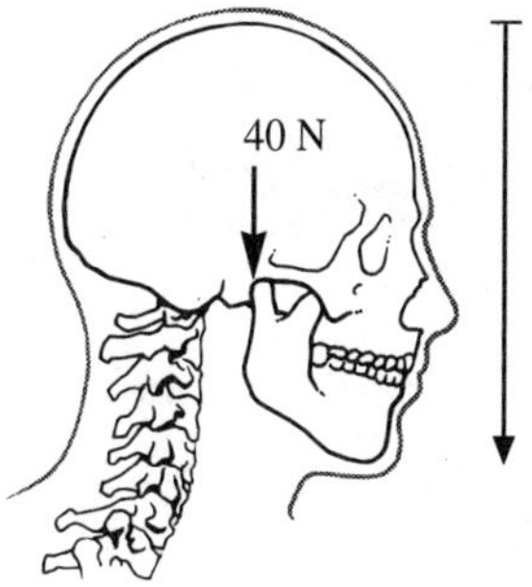

Figure 2.9 Four characteristics of a force.

2.8 MOMENT OF FORCE

So far we have only considered the tendency of a force to move a body in a straight line, a form of motion which is known as linear translation, but a force may also produce, or tend to produce, rotation of a body (Figure 2.1). In statics we must be able to predict the tendency of a body to rotate under the action of any force even though actual rotation does not occur. The tendency of a force to produce rotation about **any** point is calculated by multiplying the magnitude of the force by the perpendicular distance between the line of action of the force and the point. For example, the tendency of a weighted boot to rotate a patient's leg about the knee joint (Figure 2.10(a)) is:

Moment of force = $W \times$ distance X_1

where W is the magnitude of the gravitational force, i.e. the weight of the boot, and X_1 is the perpendicular distance between the line of action of the weight and the point which we have assumed represents the axis of the knee joint.

Perpendicular means 'at right angles to', i.e. 'at 90° to' the action line of the force. The action line of the force in this specific case is that of a weight, which **always** acts vertically downwards. The unit of the moment of a force is Nm (i.e. force × distance).

If the patient's leg is extended (Figure 2.10(b)), then, although the weight of the boot has not changed, the perpendicular distance between the point of the knee axis and the line of action of the weight has increased; consequently the moment of force is increased, so that now:

Moment of force $= W \times$ distance X_2.

Experience should suggest that the muscular effort required of a patient to hold his or her leg stationary when fully extended is greater than that required to simply allow the weighted boot to hang vertically below the axis of the knee joint (Figure 2.10(c)). In the latter case there is no moment of force because the action line of the weight now coincides with the knee axis; the perpendicular distance has been reduced to 0, and thus

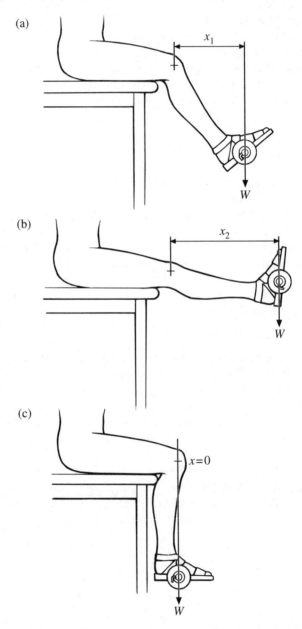

Figure 2.10 Moment of force about the knee joint due to a weighted boot.

$$\text{Moment of force} = W \times 0$$
$$= 0$$

So far only horizontal and vertical forces have been considered but forces can act in any direction in space, and techniques for resolving and combining such forces must be used to analyse many common biomechanical problems. These techniques will be introduced in Chapter 4. First, however, it will be useful to consolidate this introduction to the ideas of force, moment of force and the tendency of both of these quantities to move bodies, by examining the rules that must apply if a body remains at rest, i.e. the rules that govern a body in a state of **equilibrium**. Equilibrium is discussed in Chapter 3.

2.9 SUMMARY

Mass is a measure of the quantity of matter that a body contains and the quantity of inertia possessed by the body that resists motion, specifically acceleration. It is a property of a body that does not vary with the location of the body in the universe.

Force is a **vector** quantity, i.e. both magnitude and direction must be specified to describe a force. A vector quantity can be represented by a directed straight line drawn to scale. To fully describe a force, four characteristics must be known; its **magnitude**, **line of action**, **direction** (or **sense**) and **point of application**.

Weight is a **force** which, at or near the surface of the earth, is related to the mass of a body by the value of the acceleration due to the gravitational pull of the earth, g, where $g = 9.8$ m s^{-2}. Weight (N) = mass (kg) $\times$ 9.8 m s^{-2}. (In tutorial problems a value of $g = 10$ m s^{-2} is a suitable approximation that simplifies computation.)

Newton's three laws of motion are:

1. A body which is at rest will remain at rest unless some external force is applied to it and a body which is moving at a constant speed in a straight line will continue to do so unless some external force is applied to it. (This may also be expressed as follows: A body remains at rest or in uniform motion unless it is acted upon by an **unbalanced** set of forces.)
2. Force (N) = mass (kg) $\times$ acceleration (m s^{-2})
   i.e. $F = m \times a$
3. To every action force there is an equal and opposite reaction force.

Moment of force is the turning effect of a force about a point and is calculated by multiplying the **magnitude of the force** by the **perpendicular distance** between the line of action of the force and the point.

2.10 TUTORIAL PROBLEMS

1. With respect to the case study (Chapter 1), how would you represent the patient's weight in each of the diagrams in Figure 2.11? What is the correct SI unit for weight?

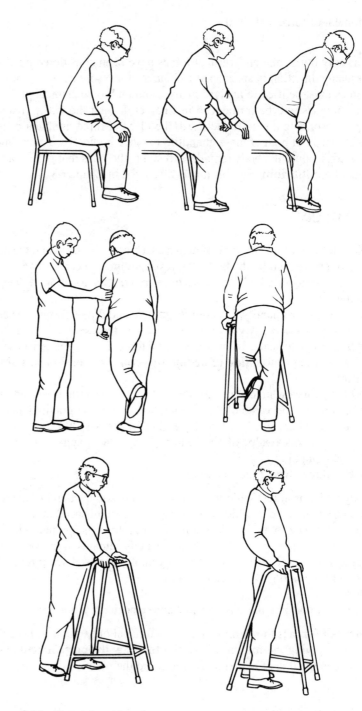

Figure 2.11 Tutorial problem 1.

2. Complete the following table.

Quantity	SI unit	Unit symbol
Length	metre	m
Mass		
Time		
Force		
Weight		

3. Weight is a vertical force. Why then is it more difficult to move a heavy object than a light object of the same volume horizontally on a perfectly smooth horizontal surface?
4. Give the weights of the following:
   (a) an adult of mass 70 kg
   (b) a human head of mass 4 kg
   (c) a textbook of mass 0.5 kg
   (d) a bar of chocolate of mass 0.1 kg
   (e) a penny coin of mass 3.56 g (1 kg = 1000 g)
5. What are the four characteristics of a force needed to fully describe it?
6. If a body which is subjected to a set of forces remains at rest, what does this tell you about the forces that are acting?
7. Explain the meaning of the statement 'force is a vector quantity'.
8. What is meant by the terms 'action force' and 'reaction force'?
9. What is meant by the term 'moment of force'?
10. When a therapist applies a force by hand to a patient's limb, the patient's limb applies an equal and oppositely directed force on the therapist's hand. Why is caution required on the part of the therapist in equating his or her effort with that made by the patient?

(See Answers section at the back of this book.)

3

3 Applying the rules for balance: equilibrium

CHAPTER OVERVIEW

Many important problems in biomechanics can be analysed by considering only the major forces that are acting in one plane (e.g. a single vertical plane or a horizontal plane or a specific anatomical plane) and by assuming that the body or body segment of interest is in a state of static equilibrium. The aim of this chapter is to introduce the concept of centre of gravity, the two essential conditions for static equilibrium and the rules for examining the mechanical stability and balance of a body in relation to its centre of gravity.

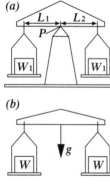

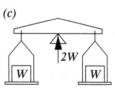

Figure 3.1 Balance and scales. (**a**) $W_1 = W_2$, the scales are balanced. (**b**) Unsupported the weights and beam will fall to earth with an acceleration of $g = 9.8$ m s^{-2}. (**c**) In equilibrium the scales are supported by a force at the pivot point equal to $2\,W$.

KEY WORDS

- Balance
- Static equilibrium
- Co-planar forces
- Principle of moments
- Centre of gravity

- Stability of equilibrium
- Line of gravity
- Base of support
- Intrinsic stability
- Extrinsic stability

3.1 STATIC EQUILIBRIUM

The term **equilibrium** has two roots: *equi* (Latin, *aequus*) meaning equal, and *librium* (Latin, *libra*) meaning balance. The sign of the zodiac Libra is a set of scales indicating balance (Figure 3.1(a)).

The concept of balance on scales is fairly straightforward; we expect that scales such as those illustrated in Figure 3.1(a) will not tip downwards at either the left hand side or the right hand side if the weights on the two pans are equal, i.e. if they are balanced.

i.e. $W_1 = W_2 = W$

This is one important aspect of equilibrium, which is analysed by the use of the concept of moment of force. If a body is at rest, i.e. if it is in **static equi-**

librium under the action of forces then any force that tends to turn the body **clockwise** about any point must be balanced by a force or set of forces tending to turn the body **counter-clockwise** about that same point.

Before examining this important principle of moments of force at more length there is another equally important rule that must apply. For a body to be in static equilibrium any force that tends to move the body in a straight line must be balanced by another force or forces that tend to move the body in the same straight line but in the **opposite** direction.

3.1.1 Balance and force

With reference to Figure 3.1(a), apart from the need for balance of the weights on either side of the pivot point, the scales as a whole must be at rest. For example, even if the weight of the beam and the pans that comprise part of the scales is ignored, the weights in each pan (W) are both tending to fall towards the centre of earth with an acceleration due to gravity, $g = 9.8$ m s^{-2} (Figure 3.1(b)). As this is not happening and they are at rest we can conclude that there is another force, acting equal and opposite to the total downward force, i.e. an upward force equal to $W + W = 2W$ (Figure 3.1(c)). This upward force is being provided at the pivot point.

Consider another example. With reference to Figure 3.2(a), if two blocks are stacked one upon the other and rest on the floor and each block is in static equilibrium then again the total downward force on each must be balanced by another force equal and opposite to the downward force.

Consider the top block. The total downward force in this case is the weight of the block W_1; consequently the lower block must be applying an upward force equal to W_1 (Figure 3.2(b)).

Now consider the lower block (Figure 3.2(c)). In this case the total downward force is its own weight, W_2, plus the downward force arising from the top block, W_1, i.e. the total downwards force is $W_1 + W_2$; as this block is at rest then the floor must be applying an upward force, R, equal and oppositely directed to $W_1 + W_2$.

A biomechanical equivalent of the previous problem would be that of equilibrium of the human body with respect to the spine (ignoring muscle and ligament forces) (Figure 3.3(a)).

The first cervical vertebra must provide an upward force to maintain the head in equilibrium (Figure 3.3(b)). The first sacral vertebra must provide an upward force to maintain the head, arms and most of the trunk in equilibrium (Figure 3.3(c)). Thus, as we proceed down the spine from the first cervical vertebra, the support provided by each vertebra to balance the superincumbent weight of body parts increases and the size of these vertebrae also increases from the cervical to the sacral region of the spine to provide the necessary strength for support of the body (Figure 3.3(d)).

Forces that tend to move a body in a straight line must be balanced if equilibrium exists, and this does not only apply to vertical forces such as those discussed so far. If a horizontal force is applied to a body and the body remains at rest there must be another horizontal force acting, equal and oppositely directed (Figure 3.4).

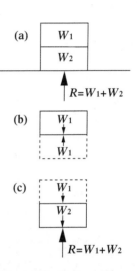

Figure 3.2 Balance of stacked weights. (**a**) Forces acting on stacked weights. (**b**) Balance of the top weight. (**c**) Balance of the bottom weight.

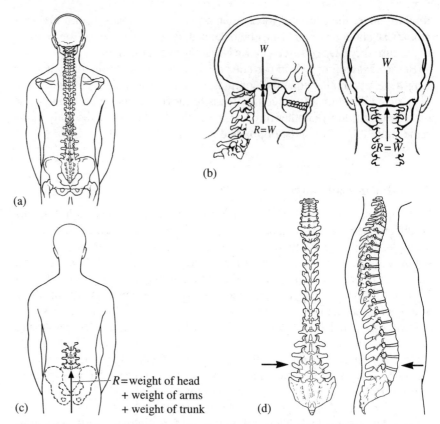

Figure 3.3 Biomechanical example of stacked weights: balance of the trunk and head. (**a**) Trunk and head: posterior view. (**b**) Balance of the head at the cervical region of the spine. (**c**) Balance of the upper body at the sacral region of the spine. (**d**) Increasing size of the vertebrae (arrows indicate position of second sacral vertebra, see p. 34).

Analysing how this oppositely directed force arises is part of the challenge of biomechanics, which can reveal some interesting aspects of functional anatomy.

3.1.2 Balance and moment of force

As stated previously, for equilibrium, any force that tends to turn a body clockwise about any point must be balanced by another force that tends to turn the body counter clockwise about the same point. An obvious point to choose to examine the requirements for balance of scales (Figure 3.1(a)), is the actual pivot point or fulcrum, point P in Figure 3.1(a). With respect to this point, P, the moment of force due to the left-hand weight, W_1, is $M_{ccw} = W_1 \times L_1$ where M_{ccw} is the counter-clockwise moment of force about point P, W_1 is the force tending to produce the turning action and L_1 is the **perpendicular** distance between point P and the line of action of the force W_1, i.e. the distance measured along a line at right angles (90°) to the line of action of the force.

The moment of force about point P due to the right-hand weight, W_2, is $M_{cw} = W_2 \times L_2$ where M_{cw} is the clockwise moment of force about point P, W_2 is

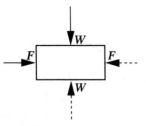

Figure 3.4 Balance of a body in the horizontal and vertical directions.

the force tending to produce the turning action and L_2 is the perpendicular distance between point P and the line of action of the force W_2.

For equilibrium: $M_{ccw} = M_{cw}$, therefore $W_1 \times L_1 = W_2 \times L_2$.

If the perpendicular distances L_1 and L_2 are equal then we can deduce that the forces W_1 and W_2 must also be equal to satisfy the above condition for equilibrium.

If the two weights are **not** equal then a state of balance can only be achieved by changing the lengths L_1 and L_2 proportionately. This effect is similar to the familiar children's seesaw (Figure 3.5).

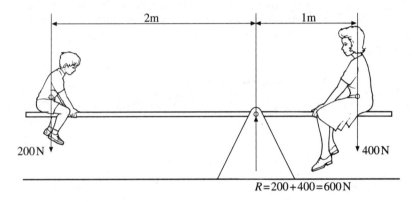

Figure 3.5   Equilibrium and the seesaw.

Thus if one child is half the weight of his partner he must position himself twice as far from the seesaw pivot point to achieve balance of the seesaw because, in this case, with reference to Figure 3.5, if the counter-clockwise moment of force is M_{ccw}, then

$$M_{ccw} = 200 \text{ N} \times 2 \text{ m}$$
$$= 400 \text{ N m}$$

and if the clockwise moment of force is M_{cw}, then

$$M_{cw} = 400 \text{ N} \times 1\text{m}$$
$$= 400 \text{ N m}$$

As $M_{ccw} = M_{cw}$, the seesaw is balanced.

Note also that to maintain equilibrium with respect to the total vertical force of 600 N acting downwards, the fulcrum must provide an equal and opposite force equivalent of 600 N upwards. We can now summarize the two conditions necessary for static equilibrium.

3.1.3   Two conditions for static equilibrium

If a body is subjected to vertical and/or horizontal forces in one plane then the following two conditions must be met if the body is to remain at rest with respect to that plane.

1. There must be no net force acting in any direction.
2. There must be no net moment of force about any point in the body, i.e. the sum of the moments of force in a clockwise direction about any point must equal the sum of the moments of force in a counter-clockwise direction about that point This requirement is referred to as the **principle of moments**.

3.2 PLANES AND CO-PLANAR FORCE SYSTEMS

In the preceding statement on the two conditions for equilibrium, it was necessary to include the phrase 'in one plane'. The term **plane** means flat. A small portion of the horizontal surface of the earth can be regarded as a plane (Figure 3.6(a)).

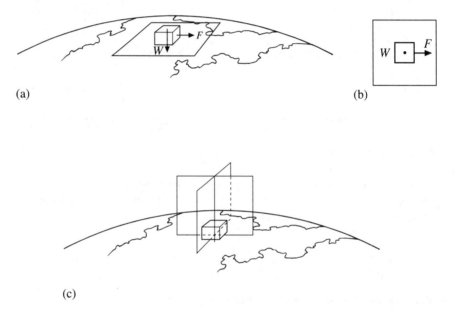

(a)   (b)

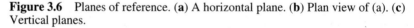

(c)

Figure 3.6   Planes of reference. (**a**) A horizontal plane. (**b**) Plan view of (a). (**c**) Vertical planes.

Consequently, when looking down on to a part of this surface, any forces acting **along** the surface would be in one plane and we would refer to a system of such forces as a co-planar force system. Gravity, however, acts vertically downwards and thus a weight could not be represented in this plane, although the position of its line could be represented by a dot on the plane (Figure 3.6(b)).

Generally in biomechanics we will be interested in viewing forces in a vertical plane, in which we can represent weight by a vertical straight line (Figure 3.6(c)).

In such a vertical plane, if the erect human body is being viewed from the front (or the back) the plane is referred to as a **frontal plane** (and sometimes the term **coronal plane** is used). When viewing the erect body from the side in a vertical plane the term **sagittal plane** is used. The erect human body can of course also be viewed from above to examine forces and force actions which are all limited to the horizontal plane; this plane is referred to as the **transverse plane**.

A convenient way of remembering these terms is to use the initial letter of each, i.e. S = side view = sagittal plane, F = front view = frontal plane and T = top view = transverse plane (Figure 3.7(a)).

If the body is rotated in space these anatomical planes rotate with the body; thus, for example, if the transverse plane is no longer horizontal it is still referred to as the transverse plane (Figure 3.7(b)).

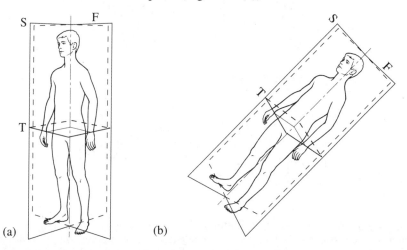

(a)   (b)

Figure 3.7 The three anatomical planes of reference. (**a**) S = side view (mid-sagittal plane); F = front view (frontal or coronal plane); T = top view (transverse or horizontal plane). (**b**) Rotation of the body in space does not change the anatomical planes of reference.

3.3   CENTRE OF GRAVITY

In the foregoing examples it has been assumed that a **line of action** of the weights can be identified and used to measure the perpendicular lengths L_1 and L_2. In fact, in Figure 3.1 the lines of action are assumed to pass through the geometrical centres of the weights. The lines of action of the forces are certainly vertical because the forces arise from the pull of gravity and the line of action of a weight is **always** vertical, acting toward the centre of the earth.

Examination of the position of the line of action of body weight in Figure 3.5 should suggest that in this case the location of this line within the body is not obvious and requires clarification; this leads us to the concept of **centre of gravity**. The centre of gravity (C of G) of an object is that point at which all of the weight of the object may be considered to be concentrated and about which the object can, **in theory**, be exactly balanced.

Thus, for example, with reference to Figures 3.8(a) and (b), if the weight of the human head (assume weight of the neck is excluded) can be balanced on the atlanto-occipital joint without the need for additional forces from muscles or lig-

LLYFRGELL COLEG MENAI LIBRARY
SAFLE FFRIDDOEDD SITE
BANGOR GWYNEDD LL57 2TP

aments then the C of G of the head must lie somewhere along the vertical line that passes through the 'pivot', i.e. the point of contact. Notice that, when viewing the head in the frontal plane (Figure 3.8(b)), the vertical line passes through the 'middle' of the head because the shape of the head is reasonably symmetrical when viewed in this direction. When viewed from the side (Figure 3.8(a)), the shape of

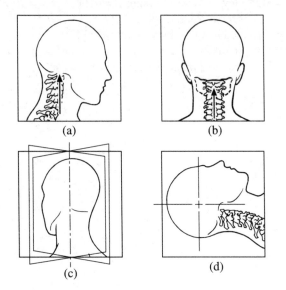

Figure 3.8 An example of the concept of centre of gravity with respect to the human head (assume weight of neck is excluded). (**a**) Line of gravity in the mid-sagittal plane. (**b**) Line of gravity in the frontal or coronal plane. (**c**) Balance must be satisfied with respect to any vertical plane that cuts the pivot point, i.e. the centre of gravity. (**d**) Centre of gravity in a sagittal plane.

the head is not symmetrical.

For convenience we usually show the position of this vertical line on one plane such as a sagittal plane or a frontal plane (Figure 3.8(a) and (b)). However, balance must be satisfied with respect to any vertical plane that cuts the pivot point (Figure 3.8(c)).

A vertical line passing through the C of G is referred to as the **line of gravity**. The weight of each particle of matter to the left of this line will produce moments of force tending to rotate the head counter-clockwise about the pivot and the weight of each particle of matter to the right of this line must produce moments of force tending to rotate the head clockwise about this point. The sum of the counter-clockwise moments must equal the sum of the clockwise moments for static equilibrium to exist.

To find the actual position of the centre of gravity along the line of gravity we could in effect attempt to balance a model of a head, say, at a different pivot point (Figure 3.8(d)), and identify a new vertical line, i.e. a new line of gravity. The centre of gravity lies on that point at which this line of gravity cuts (intersects) that found previously.

If we could now somehow insert a fulcrum into the 'head' at the position of the centre of gravity then theoretically we could balance it in any position

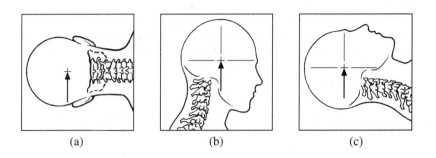

(a)   (b)   (c)

Figure 3.9 Centre of gravity and theoretical point of balance. If a fulcrum could be inserted into the head (assume weight of neck is excluded) at its centre of gravity, theoretically the head could be balanced in any position as the weight of the head will always pass through this point.

because its weight would always pass through this point (Figure 3.9).

It is important to stress that the centre of gravity of a body is a point at which we **may consider** the weight of the body to be concentrated. Of course the mass and consequently the weight is **actually** distributed throughout the body in a way dependent on the composition and structure of each part. This has important implications when we consider the posture and stability of the whole human body. For example, it is possible for the centre of gravity of a body to lie **outside** the body (Figure 3.10).

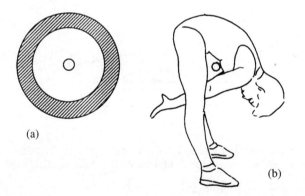

(a)

(b)

Figure 3.10 The centre of gravity (small circle) may lie outside the body. This concept is perhaps more obvious when related to an object such as a doughnut (**a**), but it can also apply to the human body, depending upon the posture adopted; compare (**b**) to (**a**).

3.3.1 Centre of gravity of the human body

The human body is not rigid and fixed and consequently there is no unique single centre of gravity for the whole body. However, if we minimize motion of the limbs and assume that our subject adopts what is referred to as a **standard anatomical position** we can determine the effective centre of gravity for the whole body for that position. For example when viewed in the frontal plane in a 'standard anatomical position' (Figure 3.11(a)), as the body is reasonably symmetrical about the midline we can envisage that it could be balanced on a pivoted board provided that the pivot was under the midline.

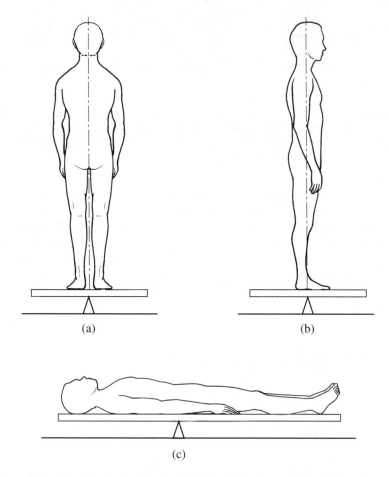

Figure 3.11 Board and pivot method of determining the position of the centre of gravity of the human body in (**a**) the frontal plane; (**b, c**) the sagittal plane.

When viewed in a sagittal plane the body is not symmetrical about a convenient midline. Nevertheless, in theory a position could be found where the body could be balanced over the pivot (Figure 3.11(b)). This would indicate a vertical line passing in front of the second sacral vertebra (see Figure 3.3(d) on p. 28 for position of this) and through the pivot point. By combining this information from the frontal and sagittal planes we can find the location of a vertical line along which the centre of gravity of the body, in this posture, must lie.

To find the position of the centre of gravity along this line, i.e. to find its **height** from, say, the soles of the feet we must now lay the body down horizontally on a pivoted board and adjust the position of either the body or the pivot to achieve balance (Figure 3.11(c)). In this position we would find that the position of the centre of gravity in a sagittal plane is in line with the second sacral vertebra.

In practice the position of the centre of gravity of the whole body is more conveniently found by what is called the board and scales method (Figure 3.12). In this method the body is still supported on a board but the board is now suspended on two supports rather than one pivot. By placing bathroom scales under these supports the force on each support is determined and by applying the principle of moments the position of the C of G is calculated.

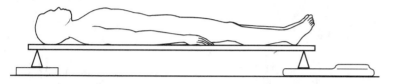

Figure 3.12   Board and scales method of determining the position of the centre of gravity of the human body.

Provided that the relative position of body parts is not varied too much the determination of the location of the centre of gravity is useful in examining a number of problems.

For example, raising both arms (Figure 3.13) will raise the position of the centre of gravity of the body a little but provided the arms are raised by equal amounts this will not affect the position of the **line** of gravity.

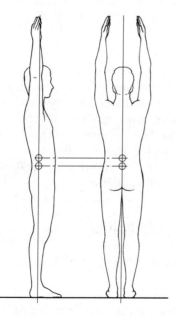

Figure 3.13   Centre of gravity and line of gravity: example 1. Raising both arms uniformly will raise the centre of gravity without altering the position of the line of gravity.

Similarly, spreading both legs apart will move the centre of gravity of the body a little in the vertical direction but will not change the position of the line of gravity (Figure 3.14 (a)). Raising only one arm or one leg will move the centre of gravity in both the vertical and horizontal directions, i.e. the position of the line of gravity will shift (Figure 3.14(b)).

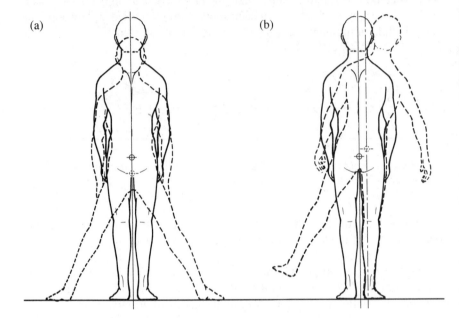

(a)   (b)

Figure 3.14 Centre of gravity and line of gravity: example 2. Raising one limb will raise the centre of gravity and move the line of gravity.

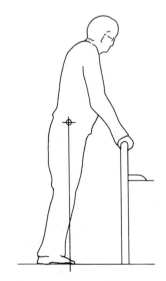

Figure 3.15 Centre of gravity and line of gravity: example 3. Line of gravity in relation to base of support.

When leaning forward, provided that the relative positions of the body parts are not changed too much from the 'anatomical position', we can assume that the position of the centre of gravity of the body is still just anterior to the second sacral vertebra. Notice, however (Figure 3.15), that the line of gravity remains vertical while the body is now inclined. In this case body weight would cause the body to topple over if some other external supporting force, such as that provided by the bath rail (Figure 3.15) were not present. This introduces us to the criteria for **stability.**

3.4   STABILITY OF EQUILIBRIUM

The classical example used to illustrate stability of equilibrium is the right circular cone (Figure 3.16).

Stable equilibrium. A body is said to be in stable equilibrium if when slightly displaced it tends to return to its original position of equilibrium under the action of the forces acting on it. Example: a cone with its base resting on a horizontal plane is in stable equilibrium; if slightly displaced it tends to return to its original position (Figure 3.16(a)).

Unstable equilibrium. A body is said to be in unstable equilibrium if when slightly displaced it tends to be further displaced by the forces acting on it. Example: a cone if placed with its vertex in contact with a horizontal plane and its axis vertical is in unstable equilibrium; if slightly displaced it will fall over (Figure 3.16(b)).

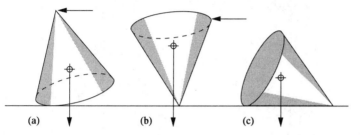

Figure 3.16 Stability of equilibrium. (**a**) Stable. (**b**) Unstable. (**c**) Neutral. The stability of a right circular cone in three positions provides the classical example of the concept of stable, unstable and neutral equilibrium.

Neutral equilibrium. A body is said to be in neutral equilibrium if when slightly displaced it remains in its new displaced position. Example: a cone if placed with its curved surface in contact with a horizontal plane is in neutral equilibrium; if slightly displaced it remains in its new position (Figure 3.16(c)).

The general rule for ensuring stability is to keep the line of gravity within the base of support. The larger the base and the lower the centre of gravity the more stable the body (Figure 3.17).

When the line of gravity lies within the base of support the weight of the body is tending to counteract any displacement, but when the line of gravity lies outside the base the weight of the body itself causes or contributes to unbalance. This applies to both inanimate objects and the human body.

The angle of tilt needed to topple a mobile hoist is one of the measures used to check the safety of this particular type of patient lifting device (Figure 3.18).

3.4.1 Intrinsic and extrinsic stability

There are two important aspects to the stability of equilibrium of the human body. The first is the requirement for **intrinsic** stability, i.e. the stability of the many segments within the body. The second is the requirement for **extrinsic** stability, i.e. the stability of the whole body with respect to its base of support.

Controlled muscular action around the joints of the spine and the lower limbs is an important feature in stabilizing the erect human body; a state of consciousness is necessary to remain upright. Nevertheless, the muscular activity is minimized if the line of action of the superincumbent weight of each

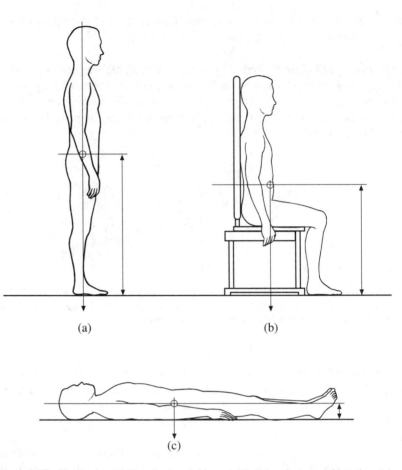

(a)   (b)

(c)

Figure 3.17 Extrinsic stability, body position and height of centre of gravity. **(a)** Standing. **(b)** Sitting. **(c)** Lying.

body segment passes through each joint that provides a skeletal fulcrum. For example, with reference to Figure 3.19, if the line of gravity of the superincumbent weight of the body above either knee joint passes behind the effective axis of rotation of the knee then the turning effect of this weight (i.e. the moment of force) will tend to flex that knee (Figure 3.19(a)). Patients with ineffective quadriceps muscles (thigh muscles) would be unable to provide the necessary muscular effort to produce balance (i.e. the necessary counter moment of force) and would consequently have an **intrinsically unstable knee**. In such cases some form of external bracing such as a caliper may be required to provide intrinsic stability (Figure 3.19(b)).

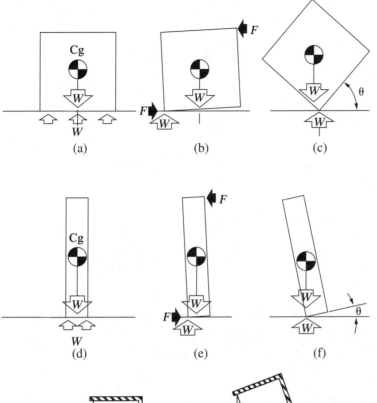

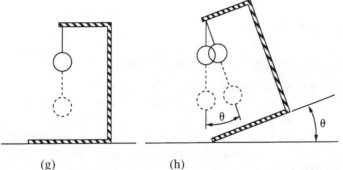

Figure 3.18 The external stability of a mobile hoist. (**a–f**) In general, the lower the C of G and the wider the base of a structure, the greater its stability. The force, *F*, required to tilt the structure will decrease as the angle of tilt increases until a position is reached where the weight of the structure itself is all that is required to complete the tilting (**c, f**). The greater the angle θ required to reach this position the more stable the structure. The upper structure (**a–c**) is more stable than the lower structure (**d–f**). NB. If the force *F* is to produce tilting without sliding then an equal and opposite force *F* must act at the point of contact with the ground, provided by friction in the case of (**b**) and (**e**). (**a–f**) It can be seen that, although the C of G of the structure moves relative to the ground with tilting, it remains in the same position relative to the structure. (**g, h**) In hoists where the body is suspended in a pendulum fashion, the patient's C of G moves relative to the structure so that at all times it is tending to be vertically below the suspension point.

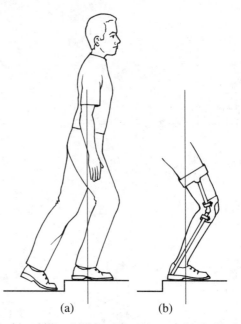

(a)   (b)

Figure 3.19 Intrinsic stability. (**a**) Line of gravity passing behind the knee joint body weight will tend to flex the knee. In a normal subject flexion will be resisted and controlled by the extensor muscles of the knee, providing **intrinsic stability**. (**b**) Intrinsic stability may be provided by external bracing such as a caliper if the extensor muscles are weak.

3.5 SUMMARY

Two conditions for static equilibrium of a body:

1. There must be **no net force** acting in any direction.
2. There must be **no net moment of force** about any point in the body, i.e. the sum of the moments of force in a clockwise direction about any point must equal the sum of the moments of force in a counter-clockwise direction about that point. This requirement is referred to as the **principle of moments**.

The **centre of gravity** (C of G) of an object is that point at which all the weight of the object may be considered to be concentrated and about which the object can, in theory, be exactly balanced.

When standing in the 'standard anatomical position' the centre of gravity of the human body lies just anterior to the second sacral vertebra.

- A body is said to be in **stable** equilibrium if, when slightly displaced, it tends to return to its original position of equilibrium under the action of the forces acting on it.
- A body is said to be in **unstable** equilibrium if, when slightly displaced, it tends to be further displaced by the forces acting on it.
- The general rule for ensuring stability is to keep the line of gravity within the base of support. The larger the base and the lower the centre of gravity the more stable the body.

Two important aspects to the stability of equilibrium of the human body are the requirements for **intrinsic** stability, i.e. the stability of the many segments within the body and the requirements for **extrinsic** stability, i.e. the stability of the whole body with respect to its base of support.

3.6   TUTORIAL PROBLEMS

1. With respect to the case study (Figure 3.20):
   (a) indicate on each of the diagrams the approximate position of the line of gravity of the patient; and
   (b) briefly comment on the stability of the subject in each position.

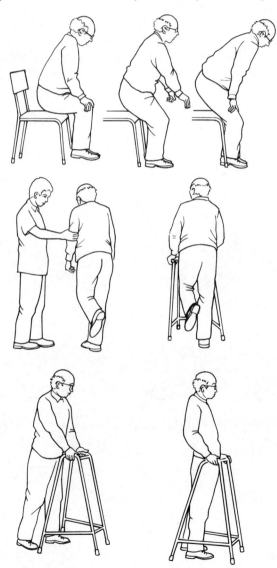

Figure 3.20   Tutorial problem 1.

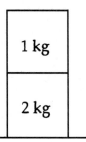

Figure 3.21 Tutorial problem 2.

2. A 1 kg mass rests on a 2 kg mass, which rests on the floor (Figure 3.21). Show the forces acting on each mass and the force acting on the floor.
3. Attempt to open a door by pushing at an area near the handle of the door and then at a point nearer to the hinged edge of the door.
   (a) In what way does the force required to open the door (i.e. the effort) change as you push closer to the hinged edge?
   (b) What mechanical principle accounts for the change in force?
4. Stand upright with your heels against a wall. Now bend forward as though to pick up an object from the floor.
   (a) What tends to happen to the balance of your body?
   (b) Explain the outcome in biomechanical terms.
5. Figure 3.22 shows the approximate position of the C of G of the trunk of a subject when leaning forward.
   (a) Show with the use of an annotated anatomical sketch the turning effect of the gravitational force at the hip joint in the sagittal plane.
   (b) Is this a clockwise or a counter-clockwise moment of force?
   (c) How could this moment of force be counter-balanced?

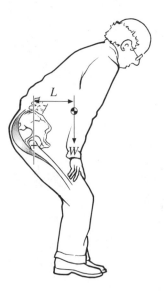

Figure 3.22 Tutorial problem 5.

(See Answers section at the back of this book.)

Solving problems with drawings: vector analysis | 4

CHAPTER OVERVIEW

Sometimes ideas are conveyed most clearly in words, sometimes in diagrams, sometimes in symbols and sometimes in numbers. One of the aims of this chapter is to extend your skill in stating and analysing problems by the use of graphical constructions and elementary mathematics in addition to words. In this chapter the concepts of concentrated external forces acting on a body, contact forces that are normal or tangential (parallel) to the surface of a body, friction and distributed forces, such as pressure, are described. The basic steps involved in simplifying and analysing a biomechanical problem are outlined with particular emphasis on graphic vector analysis, i.e. the use of scale diagrams to solve the problem of adding and subtracting a set of forces that are acting on a body at an angle to each other. Finally, the concept of the inclined plane is introduced as this provides a useful link to the topic of **machines**, which is discussed in Chapter 5.

KEY WORDS

- Free body diagram
- Tensile force, compressive force
- Concentrated force, distributed force
- Transmissibility of force
- Force vector analysis
- Space diagram, force diagram
- Composition of forces, resultant force, equilibrant force
- Parallelogram of forces, triangle of forces, polygon of forces
- Concurrency
- Contact forces, pressure, centre of pressure, friction
- Resolution of forces, component of force
- Inclined plane

4.1 STATING AND ANALYSING PROBLEMS: DIAGRAMS AND MATHEMATICS

It has already been proposed in Chapter 1 that learning involves the association of familiar and unfamiliar ideas. Graphical constructions are particularly useful for this process of association because they assist in visualizing the physical problem. A pulley can be represented by a line diagram that looks like a pulley (Figure 4.1(a)). Similarly, in biomechanics a knee can be represented by a line diagram that looks like a knee (Figure 4.1(b)). Mathematics, however, will be seen as less useful and less relevant by staff and students in some of the healthcare professions. Symbols, formulae and equations render a definite mystique and isolation to mathematics as a means of communication. This is unfortunate because without the shorthand notations of mathematics the association of more and more new ideas in biomechanics would become more and more difficult. The level of proficiency required for this text is not high and the material should not be totally new to any reader.

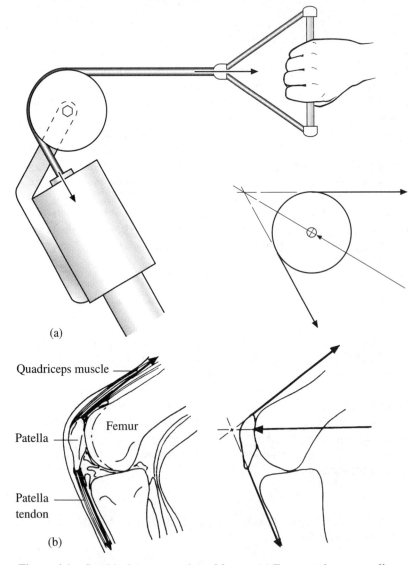

(a)

Quadriceps muscle

Femur

Patella

Patella tendon

(b)

Figure 4.1 Graphical representation of forces. (**a**) Forces acting on a pulley system. (**b**) Forces acting on the patella of the knee.

4.2 STEPS IN ANALYSING A BIOMECHANICAL PROBLEM

The basic steps involved in systematically analysing a biomechanical problem are listed in Figure 4.2. These will now be described in more detail and the opportunity taken to define or explain the terms used.

A **free body diagram** is used to clearly identify and then isolate the body (or object) or part of the body of interest. For example, to analyse the forces acting at the patellar surface of the knee in the sagittal plane (Figure 4.3), the patella is, in effect, isolated from its surrounding structures and all the external forces acting on it are represented by vectors. Bearing in mind that muscles, ligaments and tendons can only pull on a structure, then the forces acting on the patella via the attached tendons must be pulling forces; forces that pull on a body are called **tensile forces** (or tension forces) and forces that push on a body are called **compressive forces** (or compression forces). In the real situation each of these three forces will be **distributed** over a finite area; for example, tendons have a definite diameter at their point of attachment to the patella and patellofemoral contact also occurs over a finite area but by assuming that the forces are **concentrated** at specific points the effects of the forces with respect to equilibrium of the body can be determined.

In studying equilibrium, the line of action of the force is more relevant than the point of application. Neither the net (resultant) force nor the net moment of force varies with the location of the forces along their lines of action. The

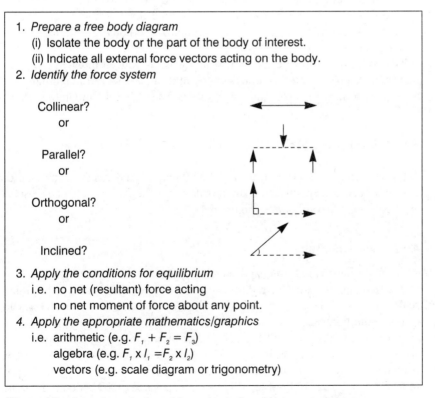

1. *Prepare a free body diagram*
   (i) Isolate the body or the part of the body of interest.
   (ii) Indicate all external force vectors acting on the body.
2. *Identify the force system*

   Collinear?
      or

   Parallel?
      or

   Orthogonal?
      or

   Inclined?
3. *Apply the conditions for equilibrium*
      i.e. no net (resultant) force acting
         no net moment of force about any point.
4. *Apply the appropriate mathematics/graphics*
      i.e. arithmetic (e.g. $F_1 + F_2 = F_3$)
         algebra (e.g. $F_1 \times l_1 = F_2 \times l_2$)
         vectors (e.g. scale diagram or trigonometry)

Figure 4.2   Steps in analysing a biomechanical problem.

principle of transmissibility states that although the **external** effect of a force on a rigid body depends upon the magnitude, direction and line of action of the force, it is independent of the point of application of the force. The **internal** effect of forces on the structure of a real deformable body does of course depend upon the site and area of distribution of the forces acting. The internal effects of forces on bodies are discussed in Chapter 6, where more precise definitions of tensile and compressive forces are also given.

In the case of the patella problem (Figure 4.3), F_1 represents the tension in the quadriceps tendon, F_2 the tension in the patellar tendon and F_3 the patellofemoral **contact force**, i.e. the force that the femur applies to the inner surface of the patella. Note that, from Newton's third law, this will be equal and opposite to the force that the patella applies to the femur. In this particular example the weight of the 'body', i.e. the patella, is ignored (the weight of the patella is very small in relation to the tendon forces, i.e. less than 1%).

These three forces acting on the patella are not **collinear**, i.e. they are not all acting in one straight line; if they were then we could use simple arithmetic to check that there is no net (resultant) force acting, a necessary condition for equilibrium. They are not **parallel**; if they were then we could again use simple arithmetic and basic algebra to check that there is no net moment of force acting about any point. They are not **orthogonal**, i.e. at 90° to each other; if they were orthogonal then we could again use arithmetic to see if all the forces acting along the y and x axes are balanced. Because the forces are **inclined**, i.e. acting at an angle to each other, and to our axes of reference, we must use some form of **vector analysis** to apply the conditions for equilibrium. We will now look at the use of graphical methods for adding or subtracting vectors.

The concept of force as a vector, which was introduced in Chapter 2, will first be restated: a **vector** is a physical quantity that has both magnitude and direction and may be represented by a directed straight line drawn to scale.

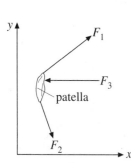

Figure 4.3 Examples of a free body diagram. Forces acting on the patella in a sagittal plane: $F_1 =$ quadriceps tendon force; $F_2 =$ patellar tendon force; $F_3 =$ patellofemoral force.

4.3 GRAPHICAL METHODS: DRAWING INSTRUMENTS

All that is required is a ruler (30 cm or 12 in) to draw and measure lines, a protractor to measure angles and a sharp pencil; a set square can also be a useful aid for drawing parallel lines (Figure 4.4).

4.3.1 Scale diagrams

After preparing a rough freehand sketch to illustrate the problem, more accurate **scale** diagrams are required for analysis. A **space diagram** is a simplified scale drawing of the part of the body of interest and this may be necessary to estimate the relative position or orientation of the forces acting on the body (Figure 4.5(a)). A force can be represented by a line whose direction corresponds to the direction of the force. The length of the line, in centimetres say, is then selected to represent the magnitude (i.e. the size) of the force in newtons; for example if 1 cm of length represents a force of 200 N then the scale is 1 cm = 200 N. In Figure 4.5(b) a free hand sketch has been used to illustrate

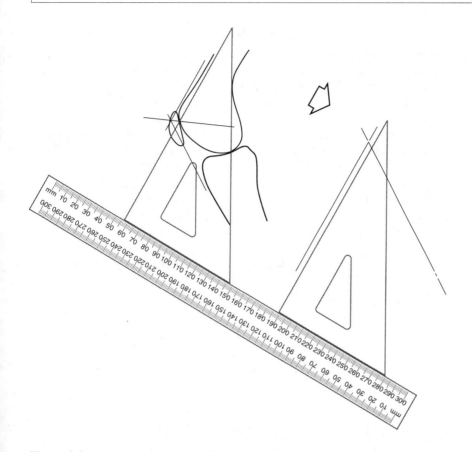

Figure 4.4 A set square as a drawing aid.

the quadriceps tendon and patellar tendon forces acting on the patella. This could represent the first stage in estimating the size of the patellofemoral contact force. The weight of the patella is ignored here because it contributes a negligible amount to the force at the patellofemoral joint. The known information is recorded on this diagram.

A separate **force diagram** is then drawn to scale (Figure 4.5(c)). The known forces are represented by lines drawn accurately in direction, using a protractor to measure angles, and the length of the lines is determined by the scale chosen; for example, if the scale is 1 cm = 100 N, then a force of 500 N will be represented by a line 5 cm long.

$$\text{If } 100 \text{ N} = 1 \text{ cm}$$
$$\text{then } 1 \text{ N} = \frac{1}{100} \text{ cm}$$
$$\text{and } 500 \text{ N} = \frac{500}{100} \text{ cm}$$
$$= 5 \text{ cm}$$

4.3.2 Composition of forces: resultant force

The term 'composition of forces' means 'composing' or adding force vectors together to determine their resultant effect. With respect to Figure 4.5, the combined effect of the two forces F_1 and F_2, i.e. the **resultant** force, F_R, can be found by constructing either a **parallelogram of forces** or a **triangle of forces**; both methods give the same result. To construct a parallelogram (Figure 4.5(c)), the vectors of the two forces are first drawn outward from the same origin, a. A parallelogram is then drawn having these two vectors as adjacent sides. The diagonal line with the same origin, a, is the **resultant** of these two forces.

Alternatively, a triangle of forces can be constructed by placing the tail of one vector at the head of the preceding one (Figure 4.5(d)). The resultant is the vector joining the tail of the first to the head of the second. A comparison of the parallelogram with the triangle in Figure 4.5 shows that triangles *abc* in both diagrams are identical. For the patella to be in equilibrium the resultant force, F_R, must be opposed by an equal and opposite force, its **equilibrant, F$_E$** (Figure 4.5(d)).

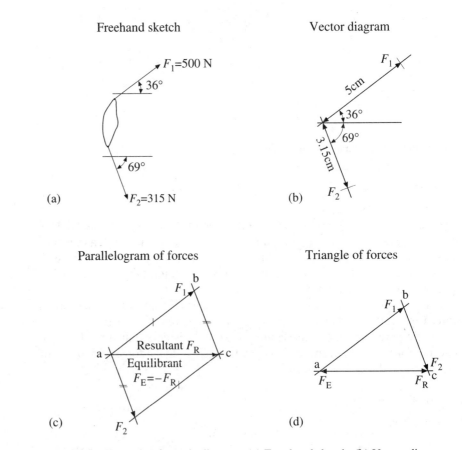

Figure 4.5 Example of a scale diagram. (**a**) Free hand sketch. (**b**) Vector diagram to scale (1 cm = 100 N). (**c**) Parallelogram of forces (resultant vector from a to c = F_R, equilibrant, $F_E = -F_R$). (**d**) Triangle of forces.

4.3.3   Polygon of forces

The method used to construct the triangle of forces can be extended as a **polygon of forces** to add three or more forces (Figure 4.6); polygon simply means 'many-sided figure'. When, as the result of the action of three or more forces, a body is in equilibrium, the resultant of all of the forces must be zero. In diagrammatic terms, **to be in equilibrium, the force polygon must close**.

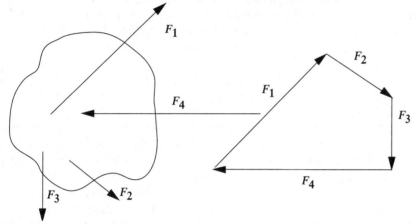

Figure 4.6   Polygon of forces.

4.3.4   Concurrency

There is a general rule that applies to a body in equilibrium under the action of three non-parallel forces and it is that the forces must be **concurrent**, i.e. their lines of action must intersect at a common point (Figure 4.7(a)). To illustrate this, assume that three forces inclined to each other do not intersect at a common point (Figure 4.7(b)). If a point where two of them intersect is selected then the third force would produce a moment of force about this point because it has a 'lever' arm with respect to this point. This would violate the conditions for equilibrium. However if the three forces do intersect at a common point then there is no net turning effect at this point.

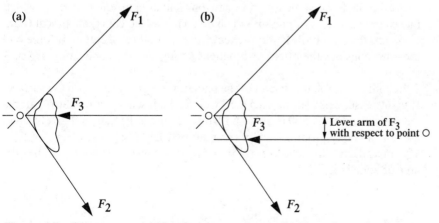

Figure 4.7   Concurrency. (**a**) Three concurrent forces. (**b**) Three forces that are not concurrent.

4.4   CONTACT FORCES

By applying this principle of concurrency to the problem of determining the contact force at the patellofemoral joint we can determine the position of the line of action of the equilibrant force on the patella in addition to its magnitude (i.e. size), orientation (i.e. angle with respect to our chosen frame of reference) and sense (i.e. direction of the arrowhead), all of which were determined from the force diagram. From this we can then deduce the 'point of application' of the equilibrant force on the patella; the equilibrant force must be a 'pushing' force on the inner surface of the patella as there is no mechanism for a 'pulling' force on the outer surface (Figure 4.7(a)). This example illustrates both the concept of the 'principle of transmissibility' of a force and the interpretation required of the analyst in examining biomechanical problems.

Naturally, in practice the so-called total **contact force** will not simply act as a concentrated force at one point but will be distributed over a finite area of the patellofemoral joint, partly in the form of a 'pressure' acting normal (that is, perpendicular) to the surface and, perhaps, in the form of a frictional force acting at a tangent to the contact surface. It is important to introduce the concepts of **pressure** as an example of a distributed force system (as distinct from the concept of concentrated force) and also to outline the main qualitative features of **friction** at this stage.

4.4.1   Pressure

Pressure is a good example of a distributed force system and is defined as **force per unit area**.

$$\text{pressure} = \frac{\text{total force}}{\text{area}}$$

$$P = \frac{F}{A}$$

In SI units force is measured in newtons and area in square metres, which makes the basic unit of pressure the N/m^2. This is also called the pascal (Pa).

As an illustration of the difference between total (concentrated) force and pressure consider the effect of a patient sitting on two contrasting surfaces (Figure 4.8).

In both cases assume that all of the patient's weight is acting on the surface. If in one case, when sitting on a hard wooden bath seat (Figure 4.8(b)), all the patient's weight, say 500 N, is supported predominantly on the relatively small area of the bony prominences of the buttocks, let us say a total area of $5 \times 10^{-3} m^2$ (50 cm^2); then the average pressure acting over the patient's skin at the area of contact is:

$$P_{\text{average}} = \frac{500}{5 \times 10^{-3}}$$
$$= 10^5 \, Nm^{-2}$$
$$= 10^5 \, Pa.$$

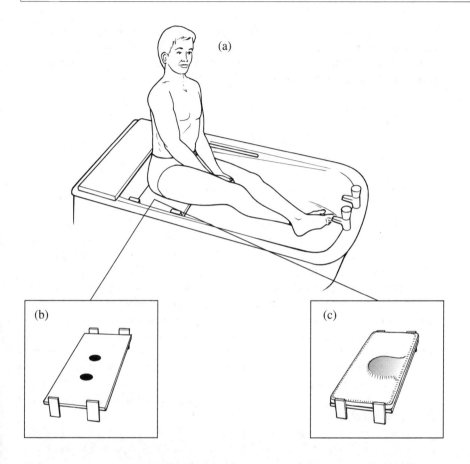

Figure 4.8 Pressure: distribution of force over area of contact. (**a**) Patient sitting on a bath seat. (**b**) Hard surface (black dots represent the two bony prominences under the buttocks pressing on a hard surface). (**c**) Soft, cushioned surface (shaded area represents where cushion is depressed).

If, in the other case, the patient is sitting on a foam cushion surface (Figure 4.8(c)), which distributes the contact force over a larger area, say $2 \times 10^{-2}\,\mathrm{m^2}$ (200 cm²) then the average pressure acting over the patient's skin at the area of contact is:

$$P_{average} = \frac{500}{2 \times 10^{-2}}$$
$$= 250 \times 10^2\,\mathrm{Nm^{-2}}$$
$$= 2.5 \times 10^4\,\mathrm{Pa.}$$

The average pressure in the case of the rigid support is, therefore, four times as great as that in the case of the cushion support, but the total downward force is the same.

i.e. $F_{total} = P \times A$

The **position** of the resultant downward force acting on the surface would be referred to as the **centre of pressure**. In general the centre of pressure is defined as the point on the surface of a body subject to external pressure at which the resultant force arising from the distributed pressure can be considered to act with the same **external** effect as the distributed pressure. The concept of centre of pressure under a patient's feet and its relationship to the patient's centre of gravity is used in analysing postural balance.

4.6.2 Friction

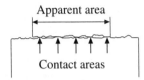

Figure 4.9 Friction: contact between surfaces.

Whenever one body slides over another frictional forces opposing the motion are developed between them. Such forces are due largely to the atomic and molecular attractive forces at the small contact areas (Figure 4.9).

Experiments with metals in contact show that when one surface is pressed against another and sliding is brought about, the enormous pressures existing at the tiny contact areas cause a kind of welding together of the two materials. With all materials in general the atoms and molecules are so close together at the contact areas that strong mutual attractive forces often pull bits of materials from one body to the other as they move along. To start a body moving is to break these bonds simultaneously, while to keep it moving is to break them smoothly and continuously. As a consequence, the deleterious effect of friction is the production of heat and wear and tear. However the role of friction in transmitting forces between bodies is an essential part of life. Friction both opposes and facilitates motion between bodies. The role of friction forces acting between the ground surface and the sole of the foot or shoe is a good example; friction is necessary to propel the body forward via the foot during the 'push-off' phase of walking and to provide a braking action via the foot during the 'heel strike' phase.

Friction may be classified as one of three kinds: sliding friction, rolling friction and fluid friction. These are discussed further in Chapters 5 and 8.

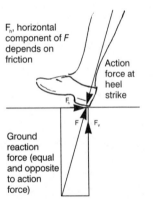

Figure 4.10 Examples of components of force. In analysing forces at heel-strike the ground reaction force, F, can be resolved into two components to assist interpretation: F_h = horizontal component of F; F_v = vertical component of F. As F_h is dependent on friction between the surfaces this resolution of a single force into two components would be useful in understanding the role of friction in this particular case.

4.5 RESOLUTION OF FORCES: COMPONENTS OF FORCE

The parallelogram of forces, the triangle of forces and the polygon of forces allow the determination of the resultant of two or more forces. In some cases it is useful to reverse this process, i.e. it is desirable to replace a single force by a pair of forces (usually at right angles to each other) that would produce the same result as the single force. Each of the two separate forces is called a **component**. When the two components are at 90° to each other they are called **rectangular** components. This technique can be used to simplify calculations of general, inclined force systems and it can also be used to aid interpretation of force systems. For example, with reference to Figure 4.10, during walking when the foot strikes the floor the force of the impact, F, acting at an angle to the surface of the floor can be more readily interpreted in terms of its two rectangular components, the vertical component, F_v, acting normal to the floor and the horizontal component, F_h, acting along the floor. If the foot is not to slip on the surface of the floor the horizontal component, F_h, must be opposed by an equal and opposite frictional force.

In this example the surface on which the force made contact was assumed to be horizontal and the force was inclined at an angle to the horizontal axis.

However the same procedure for resolving a force into two convenient components can also be applied if it is the surface that is inclined to a force that acts in a horizontal or a vertical axis. The concept of the **inclined plane** is used to analyse this general type of problem.

4.5.1 The inclined plane

If a body is placed on an inclined plane it will, in the absence of friction, accelerate down the plane under the action of its own weight, W. The weight, W, can be resolved into two components, one, F_n, normal to the inclined surface and one F_p, parallel to the inclined surface (Figure 4.11(a)).

As the body does not accelerate **into** the inclined surface then we can deduce that the surface of the incline provides a force equal and opposite to F_n. However, the component F_p provides an accelerating force acting **down** the incline (Figure 4.11(b)). If the body does not accelerate down the incline then there must be another force acting on the body equal and opposite to F_p. This may be provided by friction (Figure 4.11(c)).

The inclined plane is a good example of a method used since ancient times to raise heavy loads with a relatively small effort. It should be apparent from an examination of Figure 4.12 that, even in the absence of friction, the force E (effort) required to balance the weight W (load) on the inclined plane can be considerably less than W. This is one important characteristic of the topic referred to as **machines**, introduced in Chapter 5.

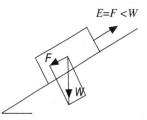

Figure 4.12 The inclined plane as a machine. Since ancient times the inclined plane has been used to raise heavy loads, W, with a relatively small effort, E, because the component of the load acting down the slope (F), which has to be overcome by the effort (E), is smaller than the load itself.

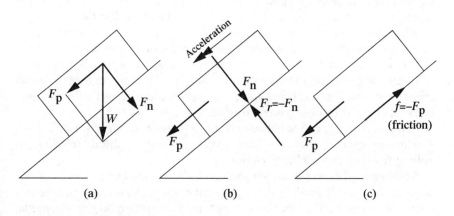

Figure 4.11 Inclined plane and components of force. (**a**) The weight, W, of the body placed on the inclined plane can be resolved into two components: F_n, normal to the surface, and F_p, parallel to the surface. (**b**) The rigid surface of the inclined plane provides a force, F_r, equal and opposite to F_n. On a perfectly smooth plane the component of force F_p would cause acceleration of the body in the direction shown. (**c**) If the body does not accelerate down the incline then a force equal and opposite to F_p must be acting: friction, f, could provide this equal and opposing force.

4.6 SUMMARY

A **free body diagram** is a procedure that aids in solving equilibrium problems. The body is 'isolated' in an attempt to identify all the possible forces that could be acting on it as a result of interacting bodies, including gravitational forces.

Forces that pull on a body are called **tensile forces** and forces that push on a body are called **compressive forces**.

The **principle of transmissibility** states that, although the external effect of a force on a rigid body depends upon the magnitude, direction and line of action of the force, it is independent of the point of application of the force.

A **space diagram** is a simplified scaled drawing of the part of the body of interest used to estimate the relative position or orientation of the forces acting on the body.

A **force diagram** is a scaled drawing in which forces, represented by vectors, may be added or subtracted.

Composition of forces is the method of determining the single resultant force that would produce the same external effect as a number of separate forces.

Resultant force is that single force that produces the same result or external effect on a body as a number of separate forces.

Equilibrant force is that single force that would maintain the static equilibrium of a body. It is equal but opposite to the resultant force.

Parallelogram of forces states that, when two forces act on a body at the same point, the resultant force will be the diagonal of a parallelogram drawn from the point of application and of which the two force vectors are sides.

When, as the result of the action of a number of forces, a body is in equilibrium, the resultant of all of the forces must be zero. In other words, to be in equilibrium, the **force polygon** must close. With three forces, such a polygon would have only three sides, i.e. it would be a **triangle of forces**.

When three non-parallel forces act upon a body in equilibrium their lines of action must intersect at a common point, the **point of concurrency**.

Pressure is normal force per unit area and is measured in pascals (i.e. Nm^{-2}).

Centre of pressure is the point on the surface of a body subject to external pressure at which the resultant force can be considered to act with the same external effect as the distributed pressure.

Friction is a force acting between surfaces that tries to stop one object from sliding over another. There are three types of friction: (a) **sliding friction**; (b) **rolling friction**; and (c) **fluid friction**.

Resolution of forces is the separation of a force into two or more components of force which produce the same result as the single force. When the two components are at 90° to each other they are called **rectangular components**.

Inclined plane is a plane at an angle to a selected axis, e.g. a plane inclined relative to a horizontal axis.

4.7 TUTORIAL PROBLEMS

1. In Figure 4.13, *F* represents the ground reaction force acting on the foot at push off.
   (a) What is meant by 'ground reaction force'?
   (b) How can a force be illustrated precisely?
   (c) How could you represent vertical and horizontal components of the action and reaction forces?
2. Diagrammatically illustrate the internal and external forces required to keep the forearm in equilibrium at the elbow joint in the position shown in Figure 4.14 for the following cases:
   (a) the line of action of the active muscle is at 90° to the horizontal ($\theta = 90°$);
   (b) the line of action of the active muscle is at 80° to the horizontal ($\theta = 80°$).

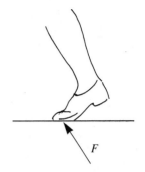

Figure 4.13   Tutorial problem 1.

Assuming that the mass of the forearm is 1 kg, determine the values of each of the forces.

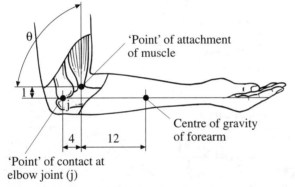

Figure 4.14   Tutorial problem 2 (all dimensions in cm).

3. Explain why the OB Help Arm (Figure 4.15), with its freely swinging support arms, permits easier horizontal movement of a supported limb than would a fixed point support.
4. Patients who suffer pain at the patellofemoral joint often complain that the pain is most intense when:
   (a) rising from a chair and
   (b) walking downstairs.
   With reference to the sketches in Figure 4.16, how would you explain this.

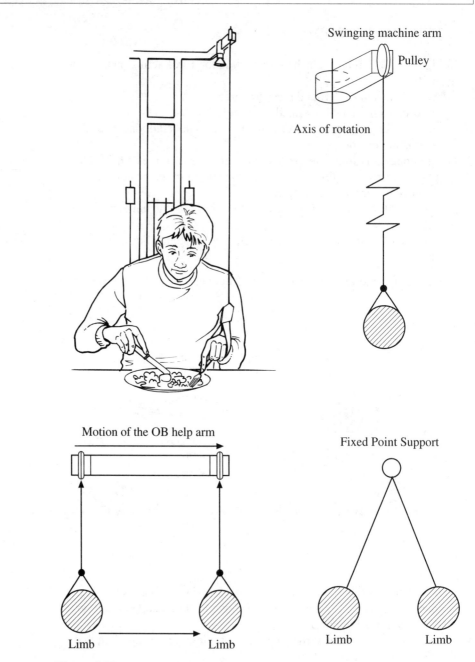

Swinging machine arm

Pulley

Axis of rotation

Motion of the OB help arm

Limb

Limb

Fixed Point Support

Limb

Limb

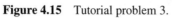

Figure 4.15 Tutorial problem 3.

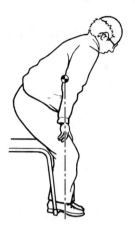 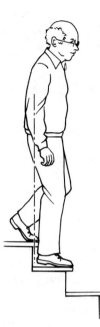

Figure 4.16   Tutorial problem 4.

(See Answers section at the back of this book.)

5 Remedial equipment: machines and mechanisms

CHAPTER OVERVIEW

Remedial equipment is commonly used in the treatment and assessment of patients. The aim of this chapter is to introduce the mechanical principles of machines, the fundamental concepts of work, power and energy and to describe the action of common mechanisms used in remedial equipment. Mechanisms include the lever, linkage, pulley, sprocket, gear, inclined plane and screw thread. The coefficient of friction is defined and machine components such as wheels, castors, brakes and bearings are discussed in relation to sliding and rolling friction. The mechanics of mobile patient hoists is used as a case study to provide an overview of conflicting mechanical design criteria. Finally the use of springs in remedial equipment is briefly described; this provides an important link to the topics of materials and structures covered in Chapter 6.

KEY WORDS

- Machine
- Mechanisms
- Torque
- Levers, linkages
- Mechanical advantage
- Velocity ratio

- Efficiency
- Friction (sliding, rolling) wheels and castors
- Pulleys
- Inclined plane, screws
- Springs

5.1 REHABILITATION MACHINES

Rehabilitation machines are devices that have been developed to provide specific movements for limbs or joints or to provide specific resistance to muscle action. Where a device is regarded as being primarily for measurement it is generally referred to as an instrument rather than a machine. Some machines of course have instruments incorporated into the device. For example the exercise machine illustrated in Figure 5.1(a) is designed to control the maximum angular speed at which a limb is moved during exercise. It does this by increasing the resistance to motion when the subject attempts to exceed the machine's pre-set speed. One of the reasons for the increasing clinical interest in this type of isokinetic (constant velocity) machine is the provision of the associated instrumentation, which provides data on the performance of the user. A full understanding of the mechanics of isokinetic devices requires an understanding of dynamics (Chapter 7), but one of the most important mechanisms in these machines is the movable lever arm (Figure 5.1(b)).

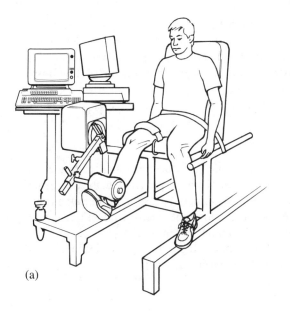

(a)

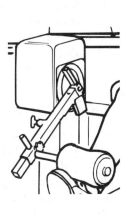

(b)

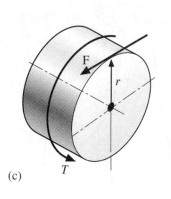

(c)

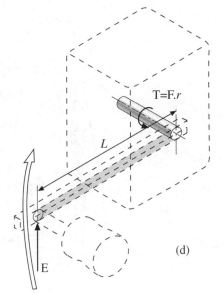

(d)

Figure 5.1 Isokinetic exercise machine.

In this discussion the term **torque** is used in relation to the resistance that acts in some machines and it is relevant to define the term here.

Torque is the same as moment of force but its use is often reserved for describing the moment of force that acts around the long axis of a shaft, i.e. torque refers to the turning or twisting action of a force, F, acting on a shaft or similar structure at a perpendicular distance, or radius, r, from the axis of rotation (Figure 5.1(c)).

Torque $= F \times r$ (N m)

If the device illustrated in Figure 5.1 provides resistance to rotation of the lever arm in the form of a known resistive torque about the axis of rotation of the lever then this torque must be equal and opposite to the moment of force applied by the limb, **provided that the axis of rotation of the limb is aligned with that of the lever**. Thus, if the limb applies an effort force, E, at a perpendicular distance, L, from the axis of rotation of the limb (Figure 5.1(d)), then

$F \times r = E \times L.$

Rehabilitation machines used by patients in occupational therapy departments tend to provide a purposeful activity for the patient, e.g. the treadle lathe (Figure 5.2) allows the patient to make something useful at the same time as providing a measurable exercise. The important mechanisms in this machine include levers and linkages, wheels and pulleys and belts.

Machines are not necessarily complicated assemblies of mechanisms; the principle of machines can be applied to a single lever.

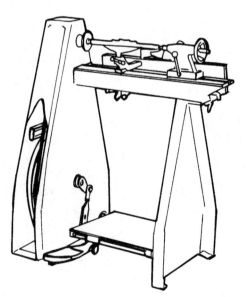

Figure 5.2 Treadle lathe.

5.2 PRINCIPLE OF MACHINES

The simple lever shown in Figure 5.3 demonstrates the basic principle common to all machines; the work (i.e. force × distance) obtained from a machine cannot exceed the work put into it and, in all practical cases, will be less because of frictional losses. The same principle applies to both manually powered and externally powered machines; however, in the latter the input will be provided by, say, electricity and not human muscle.

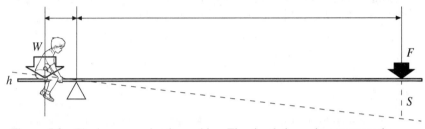

Figure 5.3 The lever as a simple machine. The simple lever demonstrates the fundamental principle of any machine, i.e. for a perfect machine, force $F \times$ distance $S =$ force $W \times$ distance h.

For example, with regard to an adjustable height chair (Figure 5.4), the user could regard the lifting mechanism as a 'black box' where work is put in at some point and less work is obtained from the box, but in a form that is more convenient to the user. In this case the therapist applies a force, an **effort**, to move a foot pedal. The effort lifts a much larger **load**, the patient's weight, but for each depression of the pedal the increase in height of the chair is small compared to the distance the pedal is depressed.

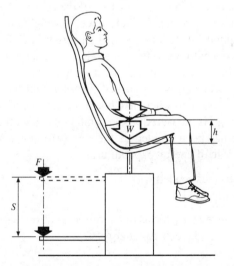

Figure 5.4 The machine as a black box. Regardless of the actual lifting mechanism employed in a hoist, the output work, $W \times h$, can never exceed the input work, $F \times S$ and in all practical cases will in fact be less because of frictional losses in the mechanism. If a force F of 120 N is used to lift a weight W of 1200 N, then for every 1 cm (h) that the weight is lifted, the force (F) must move (S) 10 cm. If it is desired to half the force F to 60 N then the stroke length S must be doubled to achieve the same lift of the weight, W.

5.3   WORK, POWER AND ENERGY

5.3.1   Work

Work is said to be done when a force, F, acting on a body, is displaced through a distance, s, in its line of action. When the force **assists** the displacement of a body then it is said that work is done **by** the force. When the force **opposes** the direction of motion it is said that work is done **against** the force. When force is measured in newtons and the displacement of the force in metres, the unit of work is defined as the joule (J), equal to one newton-metre.

> Work = force × displacement in the direction of the force
> Work = $F \times s$ (N m or J)

5.3.2   Power

Power is defined as the rate of doing work, or the rate at which work is being done. When work is measured in joules and time in seconds the unit of power is defined as the watt (W), equal to one joule per second.

$$\text{Power} = \frac{\text{work done}}{\text{time taken}} \text{ (W)}$$

5.3.3   Energy

Energy is the capacity of a body to do work. Mechanical energy may take the form of **potential energy** or **kinetic energy**. Potential energy is a measure of the capacity of a body to do work by virtue of the position (or deformation) of the body with respect to a frame of reference. A weight at the top of an exercise weight and pulley system or a stretched spring in a chest expander is an example of a device with potential energy. Kinetic energy is a measure of the capacity of a body to do work by virtue of its motion with respect to a frame of reference. A wheelchair being pushed across a floor has kinetic energy of translation and a rotating flywheel in a machine has kinetic energy of rotation. By definition energy is measured in the same units as work, i.e. in joules (J). Although power has been defined as the rate of doing work it can also be expressed as the rate of energy expenditure.

$$\text{Power} = \frac{\text{energy expended}}{\text{time taken}} \text{ (W)}$$

There are of course many forms of energy in addition to mechanical energy, such as heat energy and electrical energy.

5.3.4   The principle of conservation of energy

This allows the relationship between potential and kinetic energy to be developed and the appropriate equations are given in Chapter 7. Here it is sufficient to simply state that, in a machine, energy is neither created nor destroyed but energy can be changed from one form to another; for example, kinetic energy can be converted to heat by friction, as the act of rubbing one's hands together easily demonstrates.

5.3.5 Example

With respect to Figure 5.4 assume that the effort required by a therapist to raise a load of 800 N is 80 N. The load is raised by 1 cm when the effort moves 10 cm.

1. Calculate the work done by the therapist.
2. Calculate the power required from the therapist if it takes 0.5 s to move the foot pedal 10 cm during application of the effort.
3. Calculate the work done by the machine against the load.

Solution:
Work $=$ force $\times$ distance
Power $=$ work done/time taken

NB. Distances in centimetres must be converted to metres by multiplying by 10^{-2}.

1. Work done by therapist $=$ effort $\times$ displacement of effort
$$= 80 \times 10 \times 10^{-2}$$
$$= 8 \text{ J.}$$

2. Power required from the therapist $= \dfrac{\text{work done}}{\text{time taken}}$
$$= \dfrac{8}{0.5}$$
$$= 16 \text{ W.}$$

3. Work done against the load $=$ load $\times$ displacement of load
$$= 800 \times 1 \times 10^{-2}$$
$$= 8 \text{ J.}$$

5.4 MECHANICAL ADVANTAGE, VELOCITY RATIO AND EFFICIENCY

In the example above the work done by the therapist is equal to the work done by the machine against the load. This could only occur if there were no energy 'losses' in the machine, which is never the case. In practice the therapist would have to do additional work to overcome frictional forces acting within moving parts of the machine which always oppose motion. It should also be noted that, although the load lifted is 10 times greater than the effort required, the effort must move 10 times the distance that the load moves. In other words there is an advantage in terms of force but the cost to the therapist is the disadvantage in terms of motion. The principle of conservation of energy ensures that the therapist is not getting 'something for nothing'.

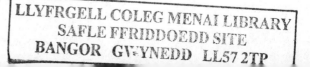
LLYFRGELL COLEG MENAI LIBRARY
SAFLE FFRIDDOEDD SITE
BANGOR GWYNEDD LL57 2TP

5.4.1 Mechanical advantage

Mechanical advantage in any machine is the ratio of the two forces, the load and the effort:

$$\text{Mechanical advantage} = \frac{\text{load}}{\text{effort.}}$$

5.4.2 Velocity ratio

Velocity ratio is the ratio of the amount of movement of the effort to the amount of movement of the load. In fact, as both the effort and load must move simultaneously, time does not enter into the calculation of velocity ratio:

$$\text{Velocity ratio} = \frac{\text{distance moved by effort}}{\text{distance moved by load.}}$$

In example 1 the therapist applied an effort of 80 N to raise a load of 800 N. In this case the mechanical advantage is 10.

$$\text{Mechanical advantage} = \frac{\text{load}}{\text{effort}}$$

$$= \frac{800}{80}$$

$$= 10.$$

The therapist moved the effort over a distance of 10 cm to raise the load by 1 cm over the same interval of time. In this case the velocity ratio is also 10.

$$\text{Velocity ratio} = \frac{\text{distance moved by effort}}{\text{distance moved by load}}$$

$$= \frac{10}{1}$$

$$= 10.$$

Note that both mechanical advantage and velocity ratio are ratios and as such have no unit of measurement.

With reference to Figure 5.4, the work done by the therapist is equal to **effort** $\times$ **distance**, $F \times S$, while the work done against the load is equal to **weight** $\times$ **distance**, $W \times h$.

By the law of conservation of energy,
input work = output work + wasted energy.

As no energy is lost in this ideal case then:

$W \times h = F \times S$
output = input,

which can be re-arranged to give:

$W/F = S/h,$

which shows that the mechanical advantage, defined as load over effort, W/F, is equal to the velocity ratio, S/h, when there are no energy losses.

The ratio of load over effort is sometimes referred to as the **actual mechanical advantage**, in which case the velocity ratio may be referred to as the **ideal mechanical advantage**. The rationale for this becomes apparent when the actual efficiency of a machine is considered. In real machines some of the input energy is usually 'lost' because of heat generated by friction between moving parts. Consequently this 'lost' energy is not available to produce an output in the form of useful work.

5.4.3 Efficiency

Efficiency of a machine is the ratio of the useful work output to the total work input. The ratio is multiplied by 100 to express efficiency as a percentage.

$$\text{Efficiency} = \frac{\text{work out}}{\text{work in}} \times 100\%$$

$$= \frac{\text{load} \times \text{distance moved by load}}{\text{effort} \times \text{distance moved by effort}} \times 100\%$$

$$= \frac{\text{actual mechanical advantage}}{\text{ideal mechanical advantage}} \times 100\%.$$

5.4.4 Example

With respect to Figure 5.4, assume that, because friction is present in the lifting device, the effort required by a therapist to raise a load of 800 N is increased from the 80 N given in example 1 to 100 N. The presence of friction cannot affect the relative amount of movement in a machine, only the forces involved, thus the load is still raised by 1 cm when the effort moves 10 cm.

1. Calculate the work done by the therapist.
2. Calculate the power required from the therapist if it takes 0.5 s to move the foot pedal 10 cm during application of the effort.
3. Calculate the work done by the machine against the load.
4. Calculate the actual mechanical advantage of the machine.
5. Calculate the velocity ratio (ideal mechanical advantage) of the machine.
6. Calculate the efficiency of the machine.

Solution:

$$\text{Work} = \text{force} \times \text{distance}$$

$$\text{Power} = \text{work done/time taken}$$

$$\text{Mechanical advantage} = \text{load/effort}$$

$$\text{Velocity ratio} = \frac{\text{displacement of effort}}{\text{displacement of load}}$$

$$\text{Efficiency} = \frac{\text{work out}}{\text{work in}} \times 100\%$$

$$= \frac{\text{mechanical advantage}}{\text{velocity ratio}} \times 100\%$$

1. Work done by therapist = effort × displacement of effort
$$= 100 \times 10 \times 10^{-2}$$
$$= 10 \text{ J}.$$

2. Power required from the therapist $= \dfrac{\text{work done}}{\text{time taken}}$

$$= \dfrac{10}{0.5}$$

$$= 20 \text{ W.}$$

3. Work done against the load $=$ load $\times$ displacement of load

$$= 800 \times 1 \times 10^{-2}$$

$$= 8 \text{ J.}$$

4. Mechanical advantage $= \dfrac{\text{load}}{\text{effort}}$

$$= \dfrac{800}{100}$$

$$= 8.$$

5. Velocity ratio $= \dfrac{\text{displacement of effort}}{\text{displacement of load}}$

$$= \dfrac{10}{1}$$

$$= 10.$$

As velocity ratio and ideal mechanical advantage are synonymous the ideal mechanical advantage is also equal to 10.

6. Efficiency $= \dfrac{\text{work out}}{\text{work in}} \times 100\%$

$$= \dfrac{\text{mechanical advantage}}{\text{velocity ratio}} \times 100\%$$

$$= \dfrac{8}{10} \times 100\%$$

$$= 80\%.$$

Therefore the machine is 80% efficient.

Using the abbreviation M.A. for mechanical advantage, the relationship between the actual mechanical advantage, the ideal mechanical advantage and efficiency can be expressed as follows:

$$\text{M.A.}_{\text{actual}} = \text{M.A.}_{\text{ideal}} \times \text{efficiency}$$

5.5 TYPES OF FRICTION: THE COEFFICIENT OF FRICTION

Whenever the surface of one body slides, or attempts to slide, over the surface of another body frictional forces opposing the relative motion are developed. All forms of friction may be classified into three kinds: sliding friction, rolling friction and fluid friction. Fluid friction is discussed in Chapter 8.

5.5.1   Sliding friction

When a force F is applied to an object of weight W in an attempt to move it across a level surface, as illustrated in Figure 5.5, the force can be increased until at a certain value the object begins to move. As the force F is increased from zero so the opposing force of friction, f, must increase to the same value to satisfy the requirements for equilibrium. In addition, in this example, for equilibrium in the vertical direction, the normal reaction force, R, must be equal to the weight of the object, W.

By relatively simple experiments, where W is in effect increased and different contact areas of objects made from the same material are used, it can be shown that the force of friction, f, that acts when motion occurs (kinetic friction) or is just about to occur (limiting static friction) is proportional to the normal reaction force, R, pressing the surfaces together, but is independent of the shape or apparent area of the surfaces in contact. Then for given surfaces

$f = \mu \times R$

where μ = the **coefficient of friction** (for given surfaces).

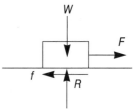

Figure 5.5   Sliding friction.

5.5.2   Example

With reference to Figure 5.6, calculate the force required to move a smooth steel block weighing 5 N across a smooth steel table top if the coefficient of sliding friction for steel on steel is 0.2.

Solution:

$$\begin{aligned} f &= \mu \times R \\ &= 0.2 \times 5 \\ &= 1\,\text{N} \end{aligned}$$

and for equilibrium, $\begin{aligned} F &= f \\ &= 1\,\text{N} \end{aligned}$

Therefore a force of 1 newton is required to initiate movement of the block.

It can be shown that the force required to just start motion is slightly greater than that required to maintain motion at a constant speed. In other words the resistance offered by **limiting static friction** is slightly greater than that offered by **kinetic friction**.

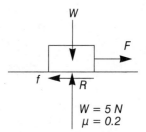

$W = 5\,\text{N}$
$\mu = 0.2$

Figure 5.6   Sliding friction (example 3).

5.5.3   Rolling friction

One of the earliest 'machines' used to move heavy objects was the roller, from which was developed the wheel and axle (Figure 5.7).

By applying a force F at the axle the effect of the force of friction, f, between the rim of the wheel and the contact surface is to cause rotation of the wheel. The force of friction is still opposing the forward motion (i.e. the translation) of the wheel and axle assembly, but the magnitude of the resistance due to rolling friction is much less than that of sliding friction.

Rolling friction is said to be due to the small relative deformation of the contact surfaces.

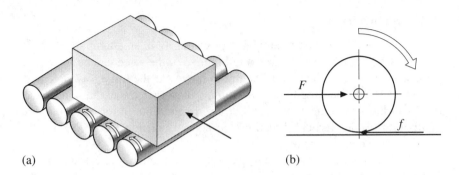

(a)   (b)

Figure 5.7 Rolling friction. **(a)** Roller. **(b)** Wheel and axle.

The form of the relationship between the force of rolling friction, f, and the normal reaction force pressing the surfaces together, R, is the same as that for sliding friction but the coefficients of rolling friction are very small.

i.e. $f = \mu \times r$

where μ = the **coefficient of rolling friction** (for given surfaces).

For example the coefficient of rolling friction for a ball-bearing on steel, μ, is 0.002, which is one-hundredth of the value for the coefficient of sliding friction for steel on steel (example 3).

5.5.4   Brakes and bearings

While friction by definition opposes motion, in another respect it also facilitates motion between bodies.

Walking is a good example of the action of friction forces in facilitating motion. In walking the foot requires an adequate foot-to-ground friction force to 'push' off at the toe region to move the body forward at the start of the stance phase of gait and also an adequate friction force at the end of the stance phase to 'brake' the forward motion of the leg as the heel strikes the ground. Water or polish on a floor diminishes the coefficient of friction between, say, shoe leather and a tiled floor, with consequences that are well known.

Rubber ferrules are provided on the bottom of walking aids to increase the friction force. Conversely, therapists use lubricants such as talcum powder to reduce friction during massage.

In a wheelchair, for example, friction prevents motion in fasteners (nuts and bolts) and secures the brakes but friction also facilitates the rolling action of the wheels.

Friction is undesirable in bearing surfaces, where the purpose of the bearing is to support and guide moving parts without resisting their motion in the desired direction. A low coefficient of friction is therefore required at the bearing surfaces of the wheel axle in wheelchairs.

Similarly, in pulley and belt systems, a high coefficient of friction is required between the belt and the grooved rim of the pulley but a low coefficient of friction is required in the bearing at the pulley axle.

5.5.5 Wheels and castors

When a wheel rolls along the surface of contact without slipping, then, during one revolution of the wheel, the axle will have moved forward by an amount equal to the circumference of the wheel (Figure 5.8).

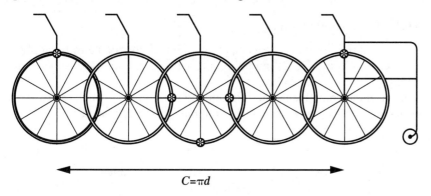

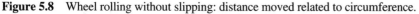

$$C = \pi d$$

Figure 5.8   Wheel rolling without slipping: distance moved related to circumference.

A wheel will move forward in a straight line unless a force is applied at an angle to the direction of progression. In a wheelchair, steering is accomplished by applying a force couple to the chair; i.e. equal and opposite forces are applied by the patient to the wheels (Figure 5.9(a)). Castors, by means of a vertical pivot (Figure 5.9(b)), are designed to follow the direction of steering by responding readily to applied torques.

(a)   (b)

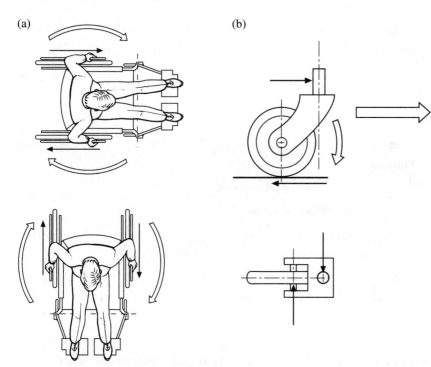

Figure 5.9   (**a, b**) Wheels and castors: steering a wheelchair.

5.6   MECHANISMS

Mechanisms such as levers, linkages, pulleys, gears and screws are used in machines to transform motion and/or force into a desired output.

5.6.1   Levers and linkages

A lever is a rigid beam pivoted at a point known as the **fulcrum**. By applying a force, the effort, at a second point, a resistive force, the load, situated at a third point is moved or balanced.

In machine components the fulcrum and the points at which the load and effort are applied have pin joints; examples of common types of lever are shown in Figure 5.10.

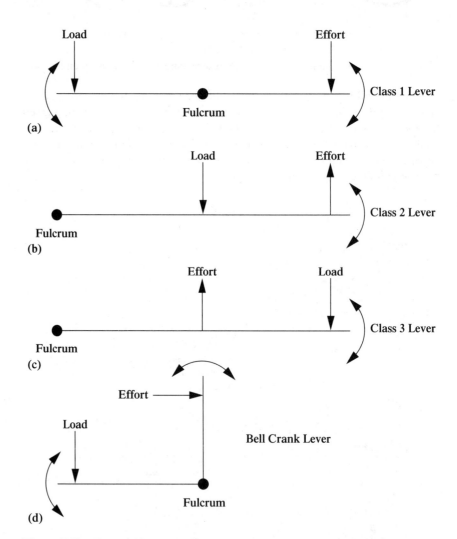

Figure 5.10   Types of lever. (**a**) Class 1 lever (also called *first order* lever). (**b**) Class 2 lever. (**c**) Class 3 lever. (**d**) Bell crank lever.

(a) Orders of lever

Three orders (or classes) of lever are referred to in engineering design depending on the arrangement of fulcrum, effort and load: a **first order lever** has the fulcrum between the load and the effort; a **second order lever** has the load between the effort and the fulcrum; a **third order lever** has the effort between the load and the fulcrum. The **bell crank lever** has the fulcrum at the junction of the two arms, which are at an angle to each other (Figure 5.10). Regardless of the type of lever used in a machine the principles of moment of force and the conditions for static equilibrium can be applied to calculate the effort required to balance a given load. In addition, the principle of machines can also be applied to determine relevant performance criteria for this 'simple' machine, e.g. mechanical advantage, velocity ratio, efficiency and so forth. In common with other mechanisms, sometimes the purpose of the machine or mechanism is only to achieve a desired motion and the only input force required is that to overcome internal resistances to motion within the machine itself.

(b) Linkages

Linkages are combinations of levers, rods and cranks that can be used to allow parallel motion, to transfer motion or to enlarge or reduce motion. For example, the parallel linkages on the seat and table units used in rehabilitation equipment, illustrated in Figure 5.11(a), ensure that the surfaces remain horizontal during height adjustment. Another example is the treadle drive in a manually operated lathe as illustrated in Figure 5.11(b), which is used to convert one type of motion into another, i.e. reciprocating motion to rotary motion.

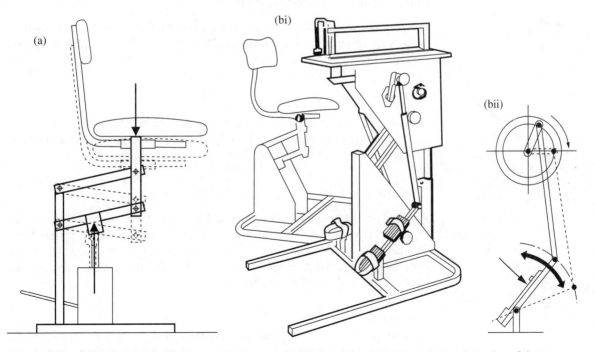

Figure 5.11 (**a, b**) Examples of levers and linkages to facilitate motion. Part bii represents the action of the arm linked to the foot pedal in part bi.

Linkages may also be used to provide a mechanical advantage, e.g. the increased clamping force in a toggle clamp or a wheelchair parking brake as illustrated in Figure 5.12.

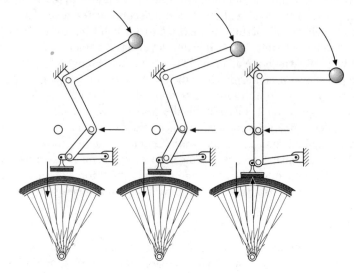

Figure 5.12 Linkages in brakes and clamps.

(a)

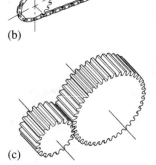

(b)

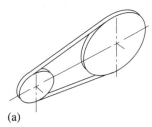

(c)

Figure 5.13 (**a–c**) Pulleys, sprockets and gears.

5.6.2 Pulleys, sprockets and gears

Motion and work can be transmitted between rotating shafts by either pulleys and belts (Figure 5.13(a)), sprockets and chains (Figure 5.13(b)), or gear wheels (Figure 5.13(c)).

Pulley and belt

Motion can be transmitted between two pulleys, which are essentially wheels with grooved rims, by a flexible belt. In general the pulleys have different diameters so that an increase or decrease in speed is achieved.

Example

The ankle rotator illustrated in Figure 5.14(a) incorporates a pulley and belt system. Assume that the input (or driver) pulley operated by a patient has a diameter of 30 cm and the output (or driven) pulley, which transmits motion to a fretsaw, has a diameter of 10 cm (Figure 5.14(b)). Calculate the velocity ratio of this pulley and belt system.

Solution:

The input pulley is three times the diameter of the output pulley. When the input makes one complete revolution the output must complete three revolutions if the belt does not slip.

(a)

(b)

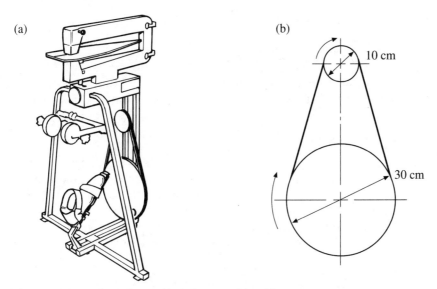

10 cm

30 cm

Figure 5.14   (**a, b**) Pulley and belt fretsaw with ankle rotator.

$$\text{velocity ratio} = \frac{\text{distance moved by effort (input)}}{\text{distance moved by load (output)}}$$

$$= \frac{1 \text{ revolution}}{3 \text{ revolutions}}$$

The velocity ratio is 1/3.

Linear velocity, angular velocity and velocity ratio

This can be derived mathematically (Chapter 7) by considering the relationship between linear and angular velocity. This shows that the instantaneous linear velocity, v, at a distance r from the centre of rotation of a body which is turning at an angular speed of n revolutions per minute is proportional to the product of n and r.

i.e. linear velocity, v, is proportional to angular speed n, $\times$ radius, r
hence v is also proportional to $n \times d$ (diameter)

which can be rearranged to give

angular speed, n, is proportional to $\dfrac{\text{linear speed, } v}{\text{diameter, } d}$

The linear speed of the belt must be constant throughout the length of the belt and hence the linear speed at the rim of each pulley is the same.
    For the two pulleys shown in Figure 5.14:

v_1 is proportional to n_1/d_1; v_2 is proportional to n_2/d_2; and $v_1 = v_2$
hence $n_1/d_1 = n_2/d_2$,

which can be rearranged to give

$$n_1 = \frac{n_2 \times d_1}{d_2}.$$

The use of single pulleys and pulley combinations in lifting devices is discussed later in the chapter.

Sprocket and chain

A chain drive, using a series of links that engage with teeth on a toothed wheel called a sprocket, can be used where a direct positive drive without slip is required (Figure 5.13(b)). The spacing of teeth on both the input and output sprockets must be equal to the spacing between links on the chain. The number of teeth of any given size and spacing that can exist on the circumference of a sprocket increases in direct proportion to the diameter of the sprocket.

$$\text{Velocity ratio} = \frac{\text{number of teeth on output sprocket } (N_2)}{\text{number of teeth on input sprocket } (N_1)}$$

$$\text{Velocity ratio} = \frac{N_2}{N_1}$$

and angular speed of output, n_2 = angular speed of input, $n_1 \times \dfrac{N_1}{N_2}$

Gears

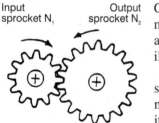

Input sprocket N_1 Output sprocket N_2

Figure 5.15 Meshed gear wheels.

Gears can also be used to transmit motion and work, without slip, between moving parts, by a series of engaging projections known as teeth. A typical arrangement of two gear wheels where the teeth are engaged or *meshed* is illustrated in Figure 5.15.

Notice that, in this case, the two wheels rotate in opposite directions. The size and spacing of teeth on both the input and output gears is equal to allow meshing. In any set of interacting gears, referred to as a gear train, the velocity ratio of the input and output shafts can be determined from the number of teeth on the input (driver) gear and the number on the output (driven) gear.

$$\text{Velocity ratio} = \frac{\text{number of teeth on output gear } (N_2)}{\text{number of teeth on input gear } (N_1)}$$

$$\text{Velocity ratio} = \frac{N_2}{N_1}$$

and angular speed of output, n_2 = angular speed of input, $n_1 \times \dfrac{N_1}{N_2}$

Gear teeth can also be machined on cylinders (to produce helical gears), conical surfaces (to produce bevel gears), shafts (to produce worm gears) and straight flat bars (to produce racks) (Figure 5.16).

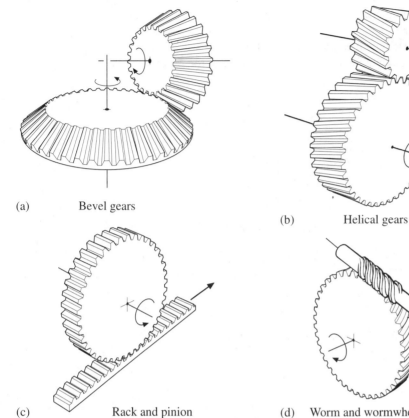

(a)   Bevel gears

(b)   Helical gears

(c)   Rack and pinion

(d)   Worm and wormwheel

Figure 5.16   Different types of gear. (**a**) Bevel gears. (**b**) Helical gears. (**c**) Rack and pinion. (**d**) Worm and wormwheel.

5.6.3   The inclined plane

As previously stated in Chapter 4 the inclined plane is a good example of a method used since ancient times to raise heavy loads with a relatively small effort. It should be apparent from an examination of Figure 5.17 that the force E (effort) required to balance the weight W (load) on the inclined plane can be considerably less than W. When viewed as a simple machine the mechanical advantage, velocity ratio and efficiency can be calculated on the basis of identifying the effort force and the load.

Consider the following example.

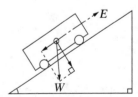

Figure 5.17   The inclined plane as a simple machine.

(a) Example

With respect to Figure 5.18(a), assume that the combined weight of a patient and wheelchair is 800 N and that a therapist is required to push the wheelchair up a ramp that has a slope of 1 in 10 (i.e. approximately 6°).

1. Calculate the minimum force that the therapist must apply to push the chair.
2. Calculate the velocity ratio of the ramp.
3. Calculate the mechanical advantage of the ramp.

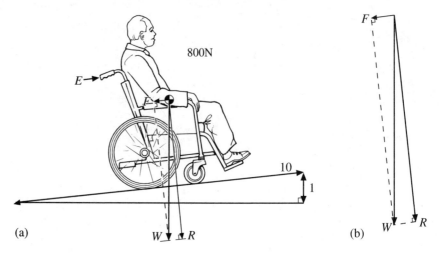

Figure 5.18 The inclined plane as a simple machine

Solution:

1. By graphic analysis (Figure 5.18(b)) the 800 N weight of the combined patient and chair can be resolved into two components, one component, R, acting perpendicular to the slope and the other component, F, acting down and parallel to the slope. It can be seen that, by measurement and calculation,

$$F = 80 \text{ N}$$

(two sides of the triangles in (a) and (b) have identical ratios of 1:10, thus $F:W$ is 1:10; if $W = 800$ N then $F = 80$ N).

For equilibrium,

effort $E = F$, therefore

$$E = 80 \text{ N}$$

The therapist must apply a force of 80 N to initiate motion up the slope.

2. To raise the load of 800 N (wheelchair and patient) through a height of 1 m the effort of 80 N (provided by the therapist) would have to travel up the slope through a distance of 10 m.

$$\text{Velocity ratio} = \frac{\text{distance moved by effort (input)}}{\text{distance moved by load (output)}}$$

$$= \frac{10}{1}$$

The velocity ratio is 10.

3. Mechanical advantage $= \dfrac{\text{load}}{\text{effort}}$

$$= \frac{800}{80}$$

$$= 10$$

The mechanical advantage is 10.

The existence of friction at the wheels would, in practice, increase the effort required of the therapist, thus reducing the efficiency of the inclined plane from the value of 100% assumed in this example.

5.6.4 The screw

The screw uses the principle of the inclined plane in that it has a projecting **thread** running along the surface of a shaft in a spiral curve; this is analogous to an inclined plane wrapped round a cylinder (Figure 5.19).

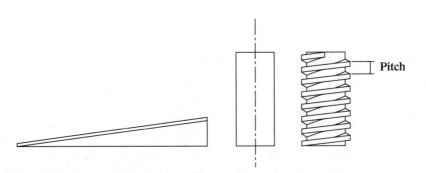

Figure 5.19   The inclined plane and the screw thread.

Although the screw is commonly used as a fastener, in machines screw threads provide important mechanisms for transmitting motion and force. The distance between two consecutive threads is called the **pitch** and one complete turn of a matching nut on a screw moves the nut parallel to the axis of the screw by a distance equal to the pitch. This mechanism can be used in machines to convert angular motion into linear motion and *vice versa* and/or to provide a mechanical advantage similar in principle to the inclined plane.

The screw jack is a common lifting mechanism (Figure 5.20).

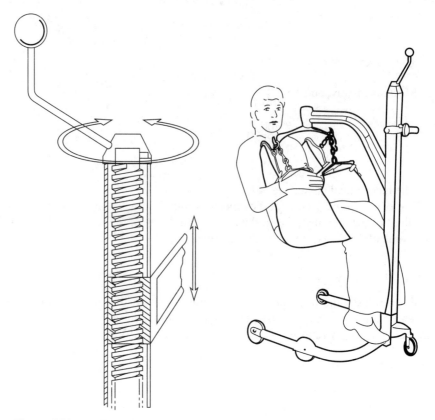

Figure 5.20 **(a, b)** Screw lifting mechanism.

5.7 PULLEYS AND LIFTING DEVICES

Pulleys and pulley combinations are used in therapy departments as simple lifting and/or support devices. For example, the fixed pulley wheel in the weight and pulley exercise equipment illustrated in Figure 5.21 simply allows weights to be raised by pulling a cord; as shown, the only advantage it offers the user is the facility to pull against the resistance of the weight in a variety of directions.

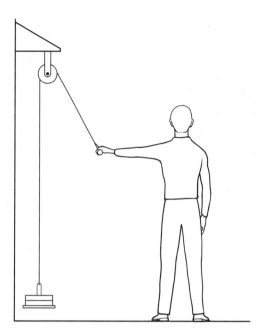

Figure 5.21   Weight and pulley.

The pulley combination illustrated in Figure 5.22 is commonly used to lift and then support a patient's limb in a particular position.

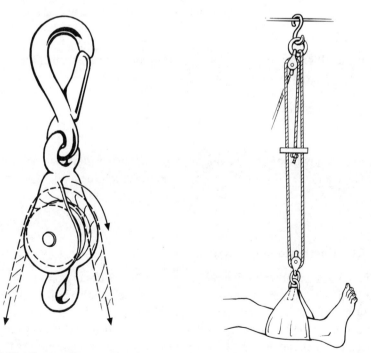

Figure 5.22   Suspension system.

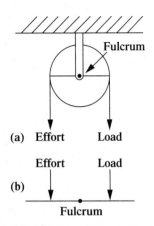

(a) Effort   Load

(b) Effort   Load

Fulcrum

Figure 5.23 **(a)** Single fixed pulley. This is analogous to a first order lever **(b)**.

The two fundamental components of pulley lifting devices are the fixed pulley (Figure 5.23) and the movable pulley (Figure 5.24).

The single fixed pulley (Figure 5.23(a)) changes the direction but not the magnitude of the relative displacement of the effort and load. It is analogous to a first order lever (Figure 5.23(b)), where the lengths of the effort and load arms are equal to the radius of the pulley. Hence,

$$\text{Velocity ratio} = \frac{\text{distance moved by the effort}}{\text{distance moved by the load}}$$

$$= 1.$$

If the pulley is mounted on frictionless bearings, which allow an efficiency of 100%, then the mechanical advantage of the system is equal to the velocity ratio of 1.

$$\text{Mechanical advantage} = \frac{\text{load}}{\text{effort}}$$

$$= 1.$$

A single movable pulley (Figure 5.24(a)) can be arranged in a form analogous to a second order lever where the load arm is equal to the radius of the pulley and the effort arm is equal to the diameter (i.e. twice the radius) of the pulley (Figure 5.24(b)). In this case:

$$\text{Velocity ratio} = \frac{\text{distance moved by the effort}}{\text{distance moved by the load}}$$

$$= 2.$$

If the efficiency of this system is 100% then the mechanical advantage is equal to the velocity ratio of 2.

$$\text{Mechanical advantage} = \frac{\text{load}}{\text{effort}}$$

$$= 2.$$

In effect, with reference to Figure 5.24, the suspension system supports half the load and the effort then only has to support half the load.

5.7.1 Combined pulley system

The system as shown in Figure 5.24(a) would be difficult to use in practice in say a patient suspension system because of the need to pull the effort in an upward direction. By adding a fixed single pulley as shown in Figure 5.23 the direction of pull can be changed while the velocity ratio and hence ideal mechanical advantage of two is retained. As there is friction in real systems the efficiency will be less than 100%. The velocity ratio will not be affected by this but the mechanical advantage will in practice be less than 2.

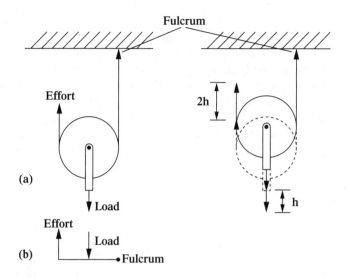
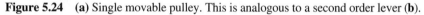

Figure 5.24 **(a)** Single movable pulley. This is analogous to a second order lever **(b)**.

5.8 HOISTS: CASE STUDY – BASIC MECHANICAL PRINCIPLES

Between the mid 1950s and the mid 1960s mobile hoists were introduced in the UK to assist in the lifting and movement of physically disabled people. The method of use of one of the early designs, imported from the USA, the Hoyer hoist, is shown in Figure 5.25(a); it can be seen that the principle is the same as that used in industrial hoists for lifting heavy machine parts (Figure 5.25(b)). The patient is supported by fabric slings and the suspension point for the slings is raised or lowered by the rotation of the jib about the top of the mast in a vertical plane. This device was manually operated and the required mechanical

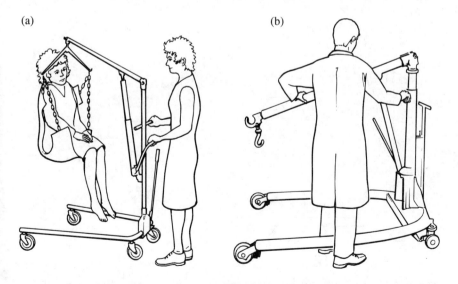
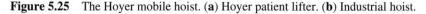

Figure 5.25 The Hoyer mobile hoist. **(a)** Hoyer patient lifter. **(b)** Industrial hoist.

advantage was achieved by the use of a hydraulic unit located between the mast and the jib. The width of the base was adjustable to allow a wide base for transportation and a narrow base for negotiating through narrow doorways.

As already stated, the basic principle common to all machines is that the work obtained from a machine cannot exceed the work put into it and, in all practical cases, will be less because of frictional losses. The same principle applies to both manually powered and externally powered hoists; however, in the latter, the input will be provided by, say, electricity and not the operator. In the case of the mobile hoist shown there is no provision of external power; the

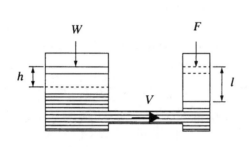

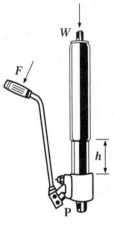

(a) (b)

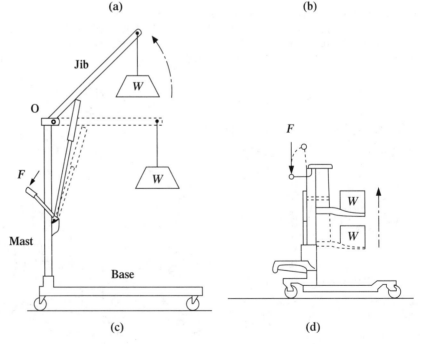

(c) (d)

Figure 5.26 Hydraulic lifting mechanisms. (**a**) Basic principle. (**b**) Example of hydraulic unit. (**c, d**) Applications.

hydraulic mechanism acts in the same manner as a manually operated lever in that the operator provides the input work.

With respect to the hydraulic system, the principle of machines still applies (Figure 5.26(a)); i.e. a small force, F, applied to a small diameter piston can raise a large weight, W, by means of a large diameter piston, but the distance that the force, F, moves is greater than the distance that the weight, W, moves. It is a property of a liquid, such as the hydraulic fluid used here, that any change in the pressure of the hydraulic fluid is transmitted undiminished to all parts of the enclosed fluid system (Pascal's principle, Chapter 8). A valve, V, will be incorporated into the hydraulic mechanism to prevent the weight falling when no force is applied to the mechanism. The actual hydraulic mechanism will be designed as a more compact unit, similar to that shown in Figure 5.26(b), where the operator applies a force to the handle of a lever, the lever operates a small plunger (piston P) and a cylinder sleeve moves relative to a shaft (h).

In the Hoyer hoists the hydraulic unit is attached across the mast and jib of the hoist and the jib rotates about the top of the mast, point O in Figure 5.26(c), to raise or lower the weight (i.e. the patient). In the Arjo-Mecanaids Pilot and the Hygiene Arjo-Mecanaids Lift Chair the hydraulic unit operated on a rigid seat attachment more directly to produce a vertical parallel motion (Figure 5.26(d)).

Again, the same basic principle of mechanical work applies if gears, pulleys or chain/sprocket mechanisms are used (Figure 5.27). In the Arjo-Mecanaids

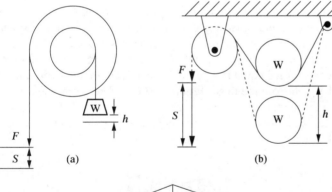

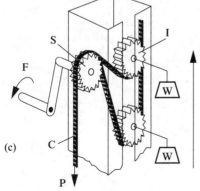

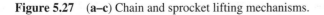

Figure 5.27 (a–c) Chain and sprocket lifting mechanisms.

Ambulift hoist (Figures 5.27(c) and 5.28), basically a sprocket wheel (I) (Figure 5.27(c)) moves up and down, within the mast, and the weight (the patient) to be raised or lowered moves in a vertical motion parallel with the sprocket wheel. The sprocket wheel is moved up and down by a roller chain (C), which is driven by an external sprocket (S).

The concept is similar to that shown in Figure 5.27(b), only the chain is not pulled but driven by the sprocket, which, in turn, is rotated by the operation of a handle.

Regardless of the actual mechanisms selected for load transmission, the limits on the load (weight) to be lifted and the force to be exerted by the operator also determine the velocity ratio, e.g. the number and length of strokes of the operating lever or wheel required to lift the patient a given height. For example, if a maximum operating force of 120 N is required to raise a load of 1200 N (120 kg) then the practical mechanical advantage in terms of force is 10:1 but, even with a perfectly efficient machine, the operating force required may make the 'effort' seem small but the increase in the number or the length of operating strokes required may be 'tiresome'. The actual mechanical advantage in terms of force will also depend upon the efficiency of the design and the materials chosen in reducing friction in the moving parts and an efficiency of the order of, say, 60% would be expected in this type of product. Ergonomic design factors such as the geometrical layout and dimensions of the operating mechanisms will influence the perceived effort of the operator.

In addition to the ergonomic requirements of the design from the point of view of both operator and patient, the engineering requirements for mechanical safety would include ensuring that the machine, as a whole and each component, can withstand maximum predicted stresses and strains (Chapter 6). To give one example, a patient suspended at the end of a jib 75 cm long would create a vertical force equal to five times his weight on the hydraulic unit if it is situated 15 cm from the mast (Figure 5.26(c)). Therefore, the actual forces transmitted throughout the machine can be well in excess of the weight being lifted and can cause bending, torsion, shear, compression and extension of the individual structures and components.

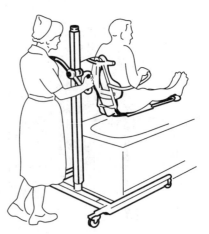

Figure 5.28 Arjo-Mechanaids Ambulift.

The overall geometry of the machine is determined by the tasks to be performed, taking account of the size and posture of the patient, the lifting height to be achieved, e.g. for bed-to-chair transfer, the environmental constraints, such as the size and clearance available for beds, chairs, baths, toilets and doorways, and the stability required for mobile devices.

In general, the lower the centre of gravity and the wider the base of the structure the greater its stability. By deliberately tilting a mobile hoist until it, in effect, falls over under its own weight, a number can be put to this stability by measuring the angle of tilt necessary for stability. In a hoist where the patient will swing in a pendulum fashion about the suspension point, stability is more complex because the patient's weight and the changing position of the patient's centre of gravity affects stability. The weight of the patient may be twice that of the hoist itself. When the base width is adjustable and the hoist jib rotates about the mast, account must be taken of the positions of these components of the hoist that cause maximum instability, as indicated in Figure 5.29. Many of the design criteria are conflicting within certain limits. For example, a small base will improve accessibility but decrease stability; small castors will improve accessibility but decrease mobility.

From the user's points of view, the overall criteria that determine the success or otherwise of each hoist are safety, acceptability to the patient and operator, ease of use and cost.

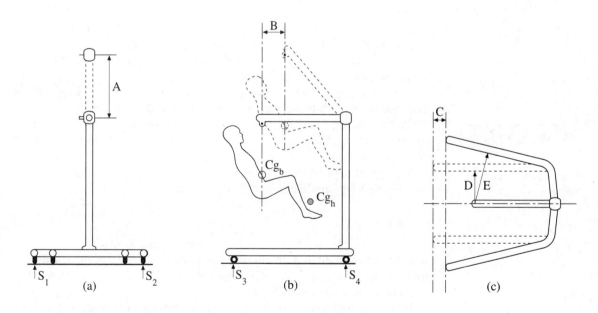

Figure 5.29 Extrinsic stability of a mobile patient hoist. (**a, b**) When the boom of a hoist is lowered by rotation about the top of the mast, this tends to increase stability with respect to sideways tilt (S_1 and S_2) and backwards tilt about S_4, but also tend to decrease stability with respect to forward tilt about S_3 because the body has moved closer to S_3 by the distance B. (**c**) If the base is widened in a similar rotational manner a similar effect occurs: sideways stability improves, forward stability decreases because of the effective displacement C.

5.9   REMEDIAL AIDS, EQUIPMENT, PROSTHESES AND ORTHOSES

The foregoing discussion, with a few exceptions, has concentrated on devices used in therapy that can be better understood by applying the basic principles of machines. There is, however, a variety of hardware used by therapists, patients and the disabled where a knowledge of mechanics is relevant. Technical aids (e.g. walking, bathing and eating aids), prostheses (e.g. artificial limbs or joints) and orthoses (e.g. splints) are examples of groups of devices where the properties of materials and structures is an important area of study. In some cases it is necessary to consider the dynamics of machines for an adequate study of its use, e.g. isokinetic exercise machines referred to at the start of this chapter. This is also true of devices that store energy, such as the flywheel used in rehabilitation machines to 'smooth out' motion.

The following brief discussion of springs is introduced here because in most therapy departments pulleys and springs are seen as basic remedial equipment. The inclusion of springs here also serves to link this chapter to the following one, which deals with materials and structures.

5.10   SPRINGS

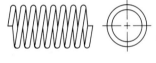

Springs are used in therapy to control movement and to apply forces. They can also be used to store energy and reduce impact forces and vibration. In the common helical coil tension spring used to provide resistance to movement during exercises (Figure 5.30) the spring consists of a continuous coil of wire wound in cylindrical fashion to form a helix.

These exercise springs, which are on average about 30 cm long, can be extended to almost twice their resting length without permanent damage. When tension forces are gradually applied from zero to some upper value to stretch the spring, the length of the spring, L, increases in direct proportion to the applied force.

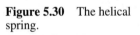

A graph of applied force, F, plotted against the corresponding extension, ΔL, reveals a straight line (Figure 5.31). Hence

Figure 5.30   The helical spring.

$$F = k \times \Delta L$$

where k is a constant of proportionality and gives a measure of the **stiffness** of the specific spring in newtons per metre (or pounds per inch in imperial units). This equation is known as **Hooke's law**.

There is a limit to the extent by which the spring can be stretched and still recover its original length when unloaded; this is known as the **elastic limit**. If an attempt is made to continue to stretch the spring beyond the elastic limit then a permanent, **plastic**, deformation will result; in this case when the spring is unloaded it will only partially recoil. To avoid this happening in therapy devices the springs have fabric tapes within the coil, which become taut when the safe limit of extension is reached.

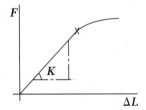

Figure 5.31   Hooke's law.

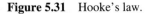

The corresponding safe maximum force at full extension is marked on a metal tab fixed to the end of the spring. It is important to realize that the number on this tab gives the resistive force, which is provided only at full extension. At any extension less than this, the resistive force provided by the spring will be proportionally less. Any attempt to extend beyond this will bring the resistive force of the cord into play in addition to that offered by the spring.

If two identical springs, i.e. springs of the same stiffness, are connected in **parallel** and stretched so that each offers a resistance, F (Figure 5.32), the effort required to stretch both is $2F$. In effect the stiffness of the device is doubled. This method of adding springs is used to increase the resistance offered by the familiar 'chest expander'.

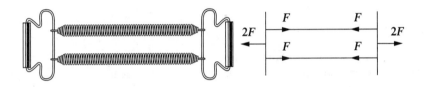

Figure 5.32 Springs in parallel.

Effort $= F + F$
$\qquad = 2F$

Hence for each centimetre of extension two identical **springs in parallel** provide **twice** the resistive force that one would provide on its own.

If two identical springs are connected in **series** and stretched (Figure 5.33) the same applied force acts all the way along the springs but the total extension of the two springs together is twice that of either of the individual springs on its own. In effect, the stiffness of the spring is halved.

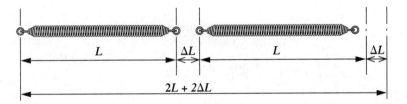

Figure 5.33 Springs in series.

$L_{total} = L + L$

$L_{total} = 2L$

In this case for each centimetre of extension of the device two identical **springs in series** provide **half** the resistive force that one would provide on its own.

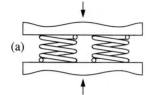

(a)

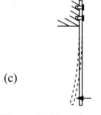

(b)

(c)

Figure 5.34 Types of spring. (**a**) Compression. (**b**) Torsion. (**c**) Leaf.

If the springs are not identical, the actual value of the spring stiffness k must be used to analyse the results of combining springs.

The above discussion of helical tension springs shows the essential elastic property of springs, but there are a variety of other forms of spring. These include compression, torsion and leaf springs (Figure 5.34).

5.11 SUMMARY

Torque refers to the turning or twisting action of a force F acting on a shaft or similar structure, at a perpendicular distance, or radius, r from the axis of rotation of the shaft.

$$\text{Torque} = F \times r \, (\text{Nm})$$

The **principle of machines** states that the work obtained from a machine cannot exceed the work put into it and, in all practical cases, will be less because of energy losses. The principle applies to all machines regardless of the source of power. By the principle of conservation of energy,

Input work = output work + wasted energy.

Work is said to be done when a force F acting on a body is displaced through a distance s along its line of action. When the force assists the displacement of a body then it is said that work is done **by** the force. When the force opposes the direction of motion it is said that work is done **against** the force.

$$\text{Work} = F \times s \, (\text{Nm or joule, J})$$

Power is the rate of doing work, or the rate of energy expenditure.

$$\text{Power (watt, W)} = \frac{\text{work done (joule)}}{\text{time taken (second)}}$$

$$\text{Power (W)} = \frac{\text{energy expended (J)}}{\text{time taken (s)}}$$

Energy is the capacity of a body to do work.

Potential energy is a measure of the capacity of a body to do work by virtue of the position (or deformation) of the body with respect to a frame of reference.

Kinetic energy is a measure of the capacity of a body to do work by virtue of the motion of the body with respect to a frame of reference.

The **principle of conservation of energy** states that in a machine, energy is neither created nor destroyed but can be changed from one form to another.

The mechanical advantage of a machine is the ratio of the two forces, the load and the effort.

$$\text{Mechanical advantage} = \frac{\text{load}}{\text{effort}}$$

Velocity ratio is the ratio of the amount of movement of the effort to the amount of movement of the load.

$$\text{Velocity ratio} = \frac{\text{distance moved by effort}}{\text{distance moved by load}}$$

The ratio of load over effort is sometimes referred to as the **actual mechanical advantage**, in which case the velocity ratio may be referred to as the **ideal mechanical advantage**.

The **efficiency** of a machine is the ratio of the useful work output to the total work input.

$$\text{Efficiency} = \frac{\text{work out}}{\text{work in}} \times 100\%$$

$$= \frac{\text{mechanical advantage}}{\text{velocity ratio}} \times 100\%$$

$$= \frac{\text{M.A.}_{\text{actual}}}{\text{M.A.}_{\text{ideal}}}$$

Friction is a force that opposes motion.

The **coefficient of friction**, μ, is defined as the ratio of the force of friction, f, that acts when motion occurs (kinetic friction) or is just about to occur (limiting static friction), to the normal reaction force, R, for a given pair of surfaces. This relationship holds for both sliding friction and rolling friction although the values for coefficients of rolling friction are generally much smaller than those for sliding friction.

$$\mu = \frac{f}{R}$$

or
$$f = \mu \times R$$

The **lever**, the **wheel** and the **inclined plane** are fundamental elements of many **mechanisms** used in rehabilitation machines to transform motion and/or force into a desired output. Such mechanisms include linkages, pulleys, gears and screws. Simple and complex machines can be viewed as 'black boxes' and the velocity ratio, mechanical advantage and efficiency can be determined experimentally. It cannot be assumed that the output of a rehabilitation machine represents the effort made by a patient unless the efficiency of the machine is known.

5.12 TUTORIAL PROBLEMS

1. Why does lengthening the handle of a tap make it easier for someone with arthritis to use?
2. An exercise weight of 2 kg mass is raised through a height of 1 m in 0.5 s. Calculate:
   (a) the work done
   (b) the average power required.
3. F_y and F_x are vertical and horizontal components of the ground reaction force F acting at heel strike. Describe how they may be related to the coefficient of friction.
4. A therapist wishes to push a patient in a wheelchair up a ramp with a gradient of 1 in 5. If the combined mass of patient and chair is 80 kg, how hard must the therapist push simply to balance the gravitational component of force parallel to the inclined surface?
   What role would friction play in assisting or resisting the therapist?
5. A smooth inclined plane can be used to provide progressive gravitational resistance to the motion of limbs during exercise. Explain, with the use of annotated diagrams, the major mechanical principles involved.
6. With reference to Figure 5.35, if the efficiency of both pulley systems illustrated is identical which system requires most effort from the patient at the position indicated?

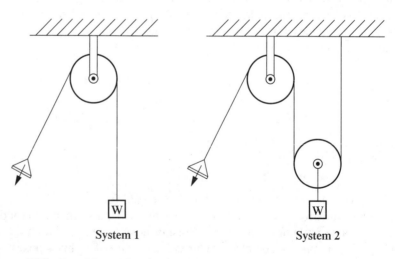

System 1   System 2

Figure 5.35 Tutorial question 6.

7. Two 30 cm long helical coil springs can be extended by equal amounts.
   The weight of each spring indicated on the metal tabs is 20 kg.
   Determine the total force in kilograms required to stretch the springs
   maximally when they are connected
   (a) in series, and
   (b) in parallel.

(See Answers section at the back of this book.)

6 Why do structures fail? Materials, human tissues and stress analysis

CHAPTER OVERVIEW

The internal effects of external forces on a solid structure depend upon:

- the distribution of the **loads** on the material of the structure
- the **stability** of the structure;
- the inherent mechanical **properties** of the material such as its **strength** and **stiffness**;
- the **size** and **shape** of the structure.

The aim of this chapter is to introduce the basic principles that are applied to the analysis of the internal effects of structures under load. This includes the use of the concepts of mechanical **stress** and **strain** to relate fundamental material properties, such as **elasticity, plasticity, viscoelasticity** and **energy storage** and **absorption**. Analysis of complex structures is simplified by identifying typical structural **elements** such as **ties, columns** and **struts, beams, shafts** and **membranes** and typical **loading patterns** such as **tension, compression, shearing, bending** and **torsion**. The chapter seeks to illustrate that the same mechanical principles used by designers to analyse man-made structures can also be applied by therapists to analyse the human body to prevent, correct or treat injuries or other musculoskeletal problems. The time-dependent behaviour of viscoelastic materials is described because of its relevance in understanding how human connective tissues respond to loading and immobilization.

KEY WORDS

- Strength, stiffness, stability
- Tension, compression, shear
- Elasticity, plasticity, viscoelasticity
- Load
- Stress, strain
- Elastic moduli

6.1 THE MECHANICS OF SOLID DEFORMABLE BODIES: CLINICAL RELEVANCE

The **mechanics of solid deformable bodies** is probably the most general title for this topic, which deals with the internal effects of externally applied forces; i.e. the events within a material or structure as it deforms under load. The principles of this branch of mechanics are applied by engineers and other specialists such as orthotists in designing and manufacturing remedial therapy aids and equipment, and orthotic devices that are worn by patients to provide physical support and to assist movement. The same mechanical principles can be applied by therapists in analysing the human body to prevent, correct or treat injuries or musculoskeletal problems that arise in other ways.

The design of any structure in remedial therapy equipment involves selecting the optimum size and shape of each part and choosing the most suitable material to meet the required function of the item within reasonable costs, taking account of the problems that will be encountered in actually manufacturing each part. The mechanical structural design criteria will include ensuring that the final product and its component parts have adequate **strength**, **stiffness** and **stability**. While therapists are unlikely to be responsible for the mechanical design of such equipment an appreciation of the design principles could be useful because they apply to all types of technical product: equipment such as exercise and rehabilitation machines, patient hoists, technical aids such as bath seats, devices worn by patients such as splints and callipers (the latter are examples of orthoses) and so forth (Figure 6.1).

With regard to the analysis of the human musculoskeletal system, because of the everyday influence of gravity on the human body, the importance of the concept of the **compressive** strength of load-bearing structures within the body is fairly obvious. Structures such as the long bones of the lower limb, the bearing surfaces of the hip and knee joints and the intervertebral discs that separate the vertebrae in the spine must have adequate strength, stiffness and stability to withstand compression (Figure 6.2(a)). Similarly, a structure whose function is to exert pulling forces, such as a muscle and a tendon, must have adequate **tensile** strength to perform the function safely (Figure 6.2(b)).

It is perhaps less obvious that compression between two solid deformable bodies can also result in disruptive tensile forces. This is certainly true in the case of the intervertebral discs, where **compressive** loads lead directly to high **circumferential tensile** forces pulling on the outer circumference of the discs (Figure 6.3(a)). It is perhaps even less obvious that compressive forces acting within, say, the hip joint can also lead to tensile failure of the articular cartilage within that joint and not compressive failure, as would be expected from a compressive force (Figure 6.3(b)).

By examining internal **stresses** and **strains**, i.e. the way in which forces and deformations are distributed within a structure, the behaviour of a structure towards external loads can be better explained (Figure 6.4).

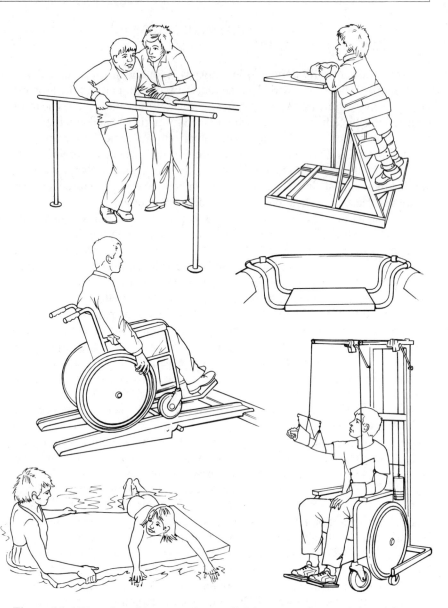

Figure 6.1 Examples of 'structures': remedial therapy equipment (adapted from Nottingham REHAB 1988 Brochure, Nottingham, UK).

The relationship between stress and strain within a structure depends upon the material of the infrastructure. From experimental work, important numerical relationships between stress and strain can be established for samples of different materials in the form of **elastic moduli**. The **modulus of elasticity**, also known as **Young's modulus**, is used to relate tensile or compressive stress and strain, and the **modulus of rigidity**, also known as the **shearing**

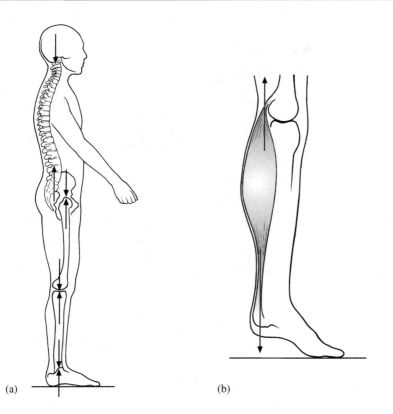

Figure 6.2 Examples of compressive and tensile forces. (**a**) Compression. (**b**) Tension.

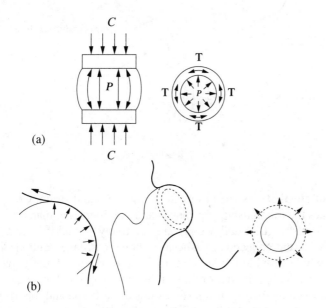

Figure 6.3 Examples of circumferential tensile forces. (**a**) Circumferential tensile force, *T*, arising from compressive forces, *C*. (**b**) Tensile forces can occur in the connective tissue.

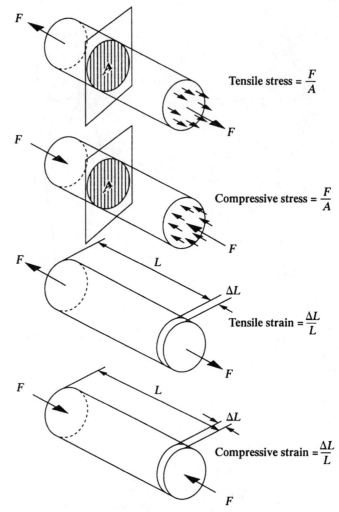

Figure 6.4 Mechanical stress and strain.

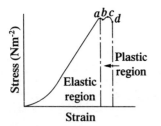

Figure 6.5 Stress–strain curve for connective tissue. a = elastic limit; b = yield point; c = ultimate (maximum) stress; d = rupture (fracture).

modulus of elasticity, is used to relate shear stress and strain. Compared to living tissues the relationships for metals and polymers (i.e. materials such as 'plastics', rubber, glass and wood) are relatively straightforward. Of the human tissues, the connective tissues, i.e. bone, cartilage, tendon, ligament and skin, which provide the supporting framework of the body, have very specific mechanical properties of direct relevance to clinical practice. The distinction between the reversible elastic extension of tissue and the irreversible plastic extension that constitutes injury is of course relevant to clinical practice and elements of the **stress–strain curves** for connective tissue are important in defining these features (Figure 6.5).

An understanding of the **viscoelastic** nature of tissues such as the ligaments and capsules that surround joints is relevant in clinical practice in understanding joint behaviour, joint protection and joint injury. Just as exercise increases the strength of muscle, active and passive mobilization of joints affects the internal structure of collagen, an important fibrous component of connective tissue, and increases the tensile strength of ligaments and capsules. Conversely, when a joint or a limb is immobilized for a reasonable length of time then the immobilization itself can result in a decrease in the strength and stiffness of the connective tissues. The concept of the time-dependent nature of viscoelastic tissues also needs to be appreciated if, during treatment, the therapist is to understand how resistance to 'stretching' varies with the speed of application of the force; for example, in vertebral manipulation during treatment for joint pain and stiffness, if the tissues are manipulated slowly they offer less resistance to stretching (Figure 6.6). At tissue interfaces, e.g. muscle–tendon–bone or ligament–bone, the speed at which the tissues are stretched during a traumatic injury will often determine which tissue ruptures.

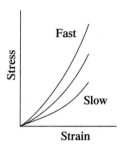

Figure 6.6 Time-dependent nature of viscoelastic tissue.

6.2 STRUCTURE, ULTRASTRUCTURE AND FUNCTION

A structure is a physical entity of a definite size and shape that usually carries a load, transmits motion or secures other structures in position. It may comprise a single material or components or composites of different materials. Even single materials vary in their **homogeneity** and **isotropy**, where a homogeneous material has a uniform distribution of the material constituents and an isotropic material has uniform mechanical properties in all directions. Bone is a good example of a composite or two-phase 'material' (collagen and hydroxyapatite) which is generally **non-homogeneous** (not homogenous) and **anisotropic** (not isotropic) (Figure 6.7).

The main mechanical criteria for effectiveness, which apply to both a man-made structure and a structure within the body, is that it must have adequate strength, stiffness and stability. In man-made structures good mechanical design involves determining the optimum size and shape and selecting the most suitable material to provide the desired function. Although man-made structures have been with us since the early history of man, the analytical approach to design really only began in the early 17th century. Fortunately, the fundamental principles that guide designers today can also be applied to the analysis of the natural structures of the human body; the latter are, however, generally much more complex than anything that designers are faced with.

Structures such as muscle are **active**, in that they can convert chemical energy into mechanical energy to generate force, whereas connective tissue structures are **passive** (Figure 6.8(a)). All living tissues can of course respond to mechanical stresses and strains by processes such as repair, which is one clear distinction from any inanimate structure. The distinction between the gross structure and the ultrastructure (or the internal structure) of a body is important in understanding its fundamental mechanical properties. For example, although passive connective tissues do not generate force by converting energy, as active muscles do, the elasticity or spring-like nature of some passive tissues is used to good effect to **store** energy (Figure 6.8(b)).

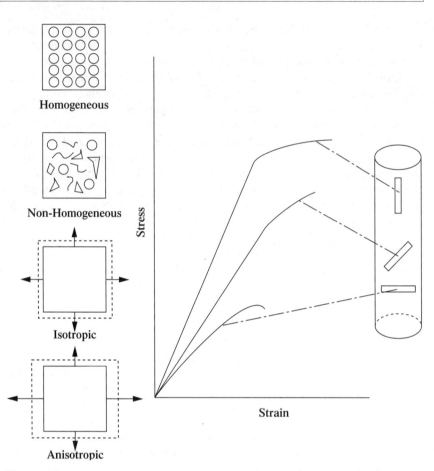

Figure 6.7 Example of a non-homogeneous and anisotropic material (bone). (Adapted from Frankel and Nordin (1980) *Basic Biomechanics of the Skeletal System*. Lea and Febiger, Philadelphia.).

Bone is found in two distinct forms in the long bones of the limbs. The shaft consists of a tube of hard **compact bone** while the ends are composed of **cancellous** or **spongy bone** covered by a shell of compact bone. The long compact bone must be stiff if it is to act as an effective lever, i.e. it requires a relatively large modulus of elasticity. Cancellous bone is more compliant than compact bone and consequently can be compressed more easily; this change in mechanical property in the structure may serve to attenuate any impulsive forces that are transmitted to the joints at the end of the long bone, by providing a shock-absorbing function (Figure 6.8(c)).

Articular cartilage, which functions as a load-bearing surface in joints, has a high fluid content, which enhances its viscoelastic properties, which in turn assists the structure to vary its response to the very variable loading that occurs during the activities of daily living; for example, different loading patterns can be expected in activities such as lying down, sitting, stair climbing, walking, running, jumping and so forth (Figure 6.8(d)).

Tendons transmit the pull of muscles to bones or fascia and most tendons pass over joints in the process. If the tendon stretches too much the contracting muscle will not move the bone effectively. However, tendons also have a relatively low shear modulus, which means that they can be flexed relatively easily in a 'pulley-cord' fashion at the appropriate site of an articulating joint (Figure 6.8(e)).

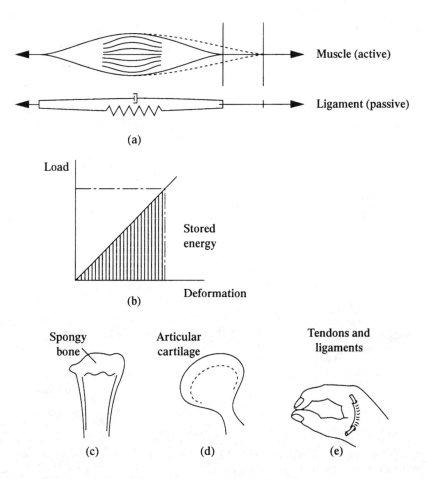

Figure 6.8 Examples of tissue structures related to function.

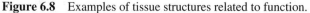

Ligaments, which stabilize joints during motion, offer more resistance to extension if loaded rapidly than if loaded slowly. Functionally, this may provide a protective mechanism to a joint by limiting its displacement during activities where rapid loading of the joint occurs (Figure 6.8(e)).

We will now look at the general principles that apply to the analysis of structures under load and define more precisely key terms that have been used in the foregoing discussion.

6.3 STRUCTURES UNDER LOAD

In developing the concepts of statics we have referred to a rigid body as one whose size and shape are not affected by the forces acting on it. It is one of a number of useful theoretical concepts that allow us to begin to examine real problems without the added complications of, for example, also dealing with the changing geometry of the body. Real solid bodies, of course, are not rigid: they deform under load. Of the three states of matter; solid, liquid and gaseous, the solid state is characterized by internal order and approximately fixed atomic positions with strong cohesive forces between molecules; these cohesive forces can be visualized as though there were springs attached to the molecules allowing some relative motion in response to external forces (Figure 6.9(a)). Liquids and gases have weak cohesive forces acting between molecules and are characterized by their inability to sustain shearing forces, i.e. they flow under the action of shearing forces (Figures 6.9(b, c)). The high liquid content of human tissues ensures a complex response of the tissues to loads (Figure 6.9(d)).

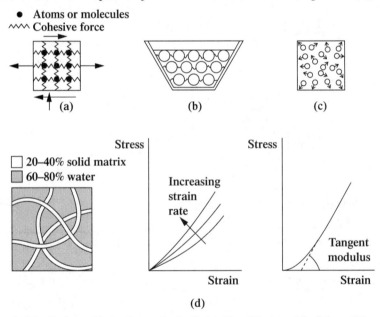

Figure 6.9 Deformable bodies under load. (**a**) Simplified model of the solid state. (**b**) Liquids. (**c**) Gases. (**d**) Articular cartilage.

6.3.1 Definition of load

There is a distinction to be made between the terms **force** and **load**. With reference to Figure 6.10, if the bodies shown are in equilibrium then at a section such as ΔL shown, which we will assume to be infinitely thin, there is no net force acting, as W and F acting in opposite directions cancel, but it is clear that there is a force effect on these sections, which can be referred to as a load. Load can be defined as the amount of force acting on **one** side of the section. In Figure 6.10(a) the load is said to be **compressive** and in Figure 6.10(b) the load is said to be **tensile**. Figure 6.10 raises another concept that was briefly referred to in Chapter 4, namely the **principle of transmissibility of force**. In

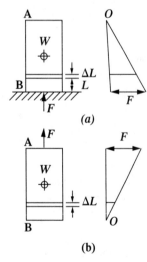

Figure 6.10 (**a**) Compressive load (load is sitting on floor). (**b**) Tensile load (load is hanging in space.)

terms of the requirements for static equilibrium the point of application of the force F required to balance W is not required to be known: it can act anywhere along the line of action of force F and W as shown in Figures 6.10(a) and (b); however, in terms of the overall **deformation** of the body and the internal stresses and strains the point of application of the force is an essential feature of the analysis. Notice that in Figure 6.10(a) compression will be maximal at the bottom of the body, at B, and there will be no compression on the top surface at A. In Figure 6.10(b) tension is a maximum at the top surface, at A, and there is no tension at the bottom surface at B.

6.3.2 Definitions of stress, strain and elastic moduli

Stress is a technical term used to express the **load per unit area** acting on a given plane within a material.

Tensile and compressive stresses are also known as **normal** stresses, i.e. they act **normal** (perpendicular) to a given plane (Figure 6.11(a, b)). The conventional symbol for both tensile and compressive stress is the Greek letter σ, sigma:

$$\sigma = \frac{\text{Load}}{\text{Area}} \left(\frac{\text{N}}{\text{m}^2} \right).$$

Shear stress (symbol τ, tau), acts **parallel** to a given plane (Figure 6.11(c)).

$$\tau = \frac{\text{Load}}{\text{Area}} \left(\frac{\text{N}}{\text{m}^2} \right).$$

Strain is a technical term used to express the **deformation** of a body (that is the change in the shape or the dimensions of a body as a ratio of the original dimensions of the body).

Tensile and compressive strains (Figure 6.11(a, b)) are **linear** strains and the conventional symbol for both is the Greek letter ϵ, epsilon.

$$\epsilon = \frac{\text{change in length } (\Delta L)}{\text{original length } (L)}$$

As linear strain, ϵ, is a ratio of two lengths it has no unit of measurement.

Shear strain (symbol γ, gamma; Figure 6.11(c)), is a measure of the change in **angle** between two lines drawn on a surface and it is measured in radians.

The **modulus of elasticity** for linear stress and strain, i.e. Young's modulus, is conventionally given the symbol E (E for elasticity). It is a measure of the stiffness of the material within the elastic region of the linear stress–strain curve (Figure 6.11(d)). Within this region the material behaves according to Hooke's law (Chapter 5): i.e. stress is proportional to strain. It should be noted that E is equal to the slope of the straight line and has the same units as stress, i.e. N m^{-2} or Pa.

$$E = \frac{\text{linear stress (N m}^{-2})}{\text{linear strain}}$$

$$E = \frac{\sigma}{\epsilon} \text{ N m}^{-2} \text{ or Pa}$$

A **tangent modulus of elasticity** may be used where a non-linear elastic response exists for any portion of the curve that approximates linearity (Figure 6.11(e)).

The **shearing modulus of elasticity** (or the modulus of rigidity), G, is the ratio of shear stress to shear strain (Figure 6.11(f)), and has the units Pa/rad or simply Pa. As explained in Chapter 7, as the radian is defined as a ratio between two lengths it has the same value in all systems of measurement and can be omitted if desired.

$$G = \frac{\text{shear stress (N m}^{-2})}{\text{shear strain}}$$

$$G = \frac{\tau}{\gamma} \, \text{N m}^{-2} \text{ or Pa}$$

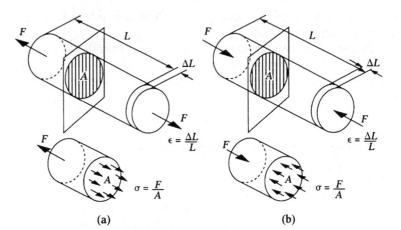

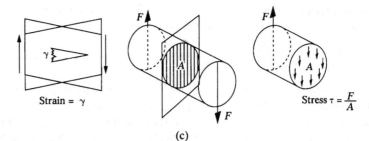

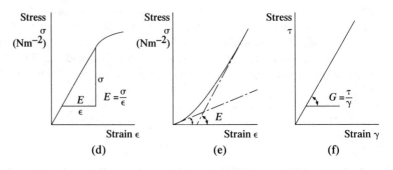

Figure 6.11 Stress, strain and elasticity. (**a**) Tensile stress and strain. (**b**) Compressive stress and strain. (**c**) Shear stress and strain. (**d**) Modulus of elasticity (E). (**e**) Tangent moduli. (**f**) Shear modulus of elasticity (G).

Real materials, particularly living tissues, respond in a very complex way to loads and to make prediction of the behaviour of a structure possible it is necessary to identify specific responses to loads or mechanical properties for simpler sections of the same material. For example, compression tests on a small cylinder of bone may be used to predict the behaviour of a whole bone to compressive loads, provided of course that the cylindrical sample is representative of the whole bone.

6.3.3 Example 1

With reference to Figure 6.12 a compressive force F of 750 N is applied to a sample of bone that has a cross-sectional area of 1 cm^2. Under this load the length, L, of the sample is decreased by 0.05%. When unloaded the sample returns to its original length, confirming that the deformation was elastic. Determine the compressive stress, strain and modulus of elasticity for the sample.

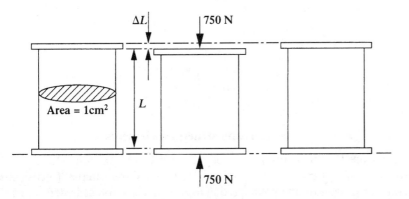

Figure 6.12 Example 1.

Solution:

$$10\ 000\ \text{cm}^2 = 1\ \text{m}^2$$

$$1\ \text{cm}^2 = \frac{1}{10\ 000}\ \text{m}^2$$

$$= 1.0 \times 10^{-4}\ \text{m}^2$$

$$\text{Stress} = \frac{\text{Load}}{\text{Area}}$$

$$= \frac{F}{A}$$

$$= \frac{750}{1.0 \times 10^{-4}}$$

$$= 7.5 \times 10^6\ \text{Pa}$$

$$\text{Strain} = \frac{\text{Change in length}}{\text{Original length}}$$

$$= \frac{\Delta L}{L}$$

$$= \frac{0.05}{100}$$

$$= 0.0005$$

$$= 5 \times 10^{-4}$$

(NB. When strain is expressed as a percentage change, as it is in this problem, this is the change in length per 100 units of the original length; i.e. 0.05% is 0.05 m per 100 m or 0.05 mm per 100 mm or 0.05 in per 100 in, etc.)

Assuming a linear stress–strain curve, then:

$$\text{Modulus of elasticity, } E = \frac{\text{stress}}{\text{strain}}$$

$$= \frac{\sigma}{\epsilon}$$

$$= \frac{7.5 \times 10^6}{5.0 \times 10^{-4}}$$

$$= 1.5 \times 10^{10} \text{ Pa}$$

6.3.4 Typical load patterns and structural elements

Having used the concepts of free body diagrams and equilibrium to isolate the structure of particular interest and to determine all the external forces acting upon it we can now attempt to predict the effect of the forces in deforming the structure. Real structures can of course be very complicated in terms of size and shape and to assist in analysis it is common practice to attempt to identify typical loading patterns that tend to stretch, compress, shear, bend or twist sections of the structure (Figure 6.13).

Tension and compression occurs when equal and opposite forces act **in line** across a section of a structure (Figure 6.13(a)).

Shearing occurs when equal and opposite forces are **out of line** across a section of a structure (Figure 6.13(b)).

Bending of structures occurs when forces produce equal and opposite **moment actions** about a section of a structure. If two equal and opposite moments of force are applied to the ends of a structural element called a **beam**, which may be in the form of a horizontal bar, then bending of the beam will occur. The internal effect on the beam is to stretch the outer edge of the beam and to compress the inner edge. Between the two edges is a line or axis that is neither stretched nor compressed this is called the **neutral axis** of the beam. In a linear elastic material the stress increases linearly from zero at the neutral axis to a maximum at each surface (Figure 6.13(c)).

In most cases beams are also subjected to **vertical shearing forces** because of the distribution of forces along the beam in the form of loads and reaction forces at the points of support of the beam (Figure 6.13(d)). In these cases although there is no tensile or compressive stress acting along the neutral axis there is a shear stress acting **along** this axis, which the beam material must resist. These effects can perhaps be better visualized by considering the beam as though it was constructed from freely moving individual layers, similar to a pack of cards. If this 'pack of cards' is flexed then the individual layers will, in effect, slide relative to each other, essentially keeping their same lengths. If, however, the individual layers or cards were 'glued' together then, in addition to the stretching and compression that would take place at the two respective outer edges to achieve the final shape of the 'beam', horizontal shearing forces would also act to resist sliding between the layers (Figure 6.13(e)).

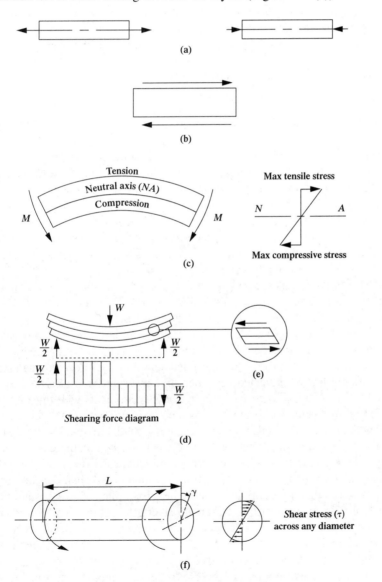

Figure 6.13 Typical load patterns. (**a**) Tension and compression. (**b**) Shearing. (**c**) Bending (of a beam). (**d, e**) Vertical shearing force; (**f**) Torsion.

Torsion of a structure occurs because of the moment action of a force about the **longitudinal** axis of the structure. If torque is applied about the longitudinal axis at the opposite ends of, say, a shaft, then twisting will occur. In this case shearing stresses act on planes that are **perpendicular** to the longitudinal axis. In a circular cross-section of a shaft of linearly elastic material, while the shear stress is distributed across the entire section, maximum shear stress acts at the outer edge of the shaft (Figure 6.13(f)).

Structural elements such as **ties**, which carry tensile loads, **columns, pillars** and **struts**, which carry compressive loads, and **beams** and **cantilevers**, which carry bending loads, are used in design analysis; the cantilever is a beam that is fixed or supported at one end only. A **shaft** is a common structural element which may be subjected to torque, and a **membrane** is another useful element, which can be used to analyse thin shell-like structures such as hollow, thin-walled cylinders or spheres, or indeed strapping and the fabric slings used in patient hoists (Figure 6.14).

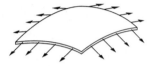

Figure 6.14 Membranes.

6.4   THE TENSILE TEST

Strength, stiffness and stability are the performance criteria for any structure that must carry a load. A structure may fail by **fracturing**, by **deforming** too much or by **buckling**, the last being one measure of instability. Before looking at some of the factors that influence the optimum size, shape and form of a structure to withstand either static or dynamic loads it is important to examine the fundamental mechanical properties of strength and stiffness of materials. These properties are usually determined from tensile tests on carefully selected samples of the material.

The simple 'tie' under tension provides a good example of the way that linear stress and strain can be related to material properties. Figure 6.15(a) shows the relationship between tensile force and the resulting extension of a metal rod in the form of a load–deformation graph. Initially the material behaves elastically, i.e. if the force is removed before point *a*, a point referred to as the **elastic limit**, the rod returns to its original length. If the force–extension graph is a straight line as indicated here then, like a spring, the rod is said to obey Hooke's law. If the force is increased beyond point *a*, **yielding** or **plastic** deformation begins, i.e. if the force is removed after point *a* the length of the rod will have been permanently increased by a small amount. In **ductile** materials, i.e. materials that deform extensively before fracture, there is a point just beyond the elastic limit where deformation increases without any increase in force and this is defined as the **yield point**, point *b*. Many materials do not possess a well defined yield point. The highest force the rod can sustain before fracture is termed the **ultimate tensile strength**, point *c*. Failure occurs at point *d*. In practical tensile tests it is possible to reduce the force as the test proceeds beyond point *c* and still cause failure. This is because although the force is slightly reduced, the internal **stress** is not; in ductile materials 'necking' occurs at the fracture site, i.e. the cross-sectional area of the rod begins to decrease before fracture and the force required to generate internal stresses decreases as the area decreases (force = stress × area).

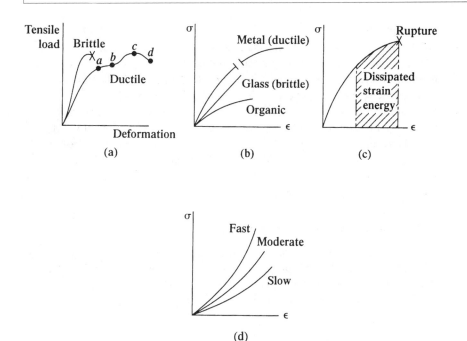

Figure 6.15 Load–deformation and stress–strain diagrams for materials in tension. (**a**) Load–deformation. (**b**) Idealized stress–strain diagrams for distinct classes of material. (**c**) Strain energy. (**d**) Strain rate.

The behaviour of the rod depends, of course, on its size. If we double the cross-sectional area this is similar to placing two springs in **parallel** (Chapter 5) and we would have to double the force to obtain an extension the same as that which would be produced in one spring. Similarly, doubling the cross-sectional area of the rod would require double the force to produce an extension the same as that which would be produced in one rod. Doubling the **length** of the rod is like having two springs in **series** and consequently the total extension for a given force is twice that which the same force would produce in a single rod. The problem of the size of the sample of material under test, e.g. the size of the rod, is overcome by plotting **stress** against **strain** instead of load against extension (Figure 6.15(b)). The shape of the graph or curve is generally similar to the load–extension graph for the particular material; examples of the general shape of curves for ductile, brittle and organic materials is shown in Figure 6.15(b). **Brittle** materials such as cast iron and glass are not capable of withstanding large strains whereas ductile materials such as mild steel and aluminium are. The area under a stress–strain curve is a measure of the energy absorption capacity or **toughness** of a material and is closely related to the concepts of ductility and brittleness (Figure 6.15(c)).

6.4.1 Factor of safety

In the design of a tie, if the maximum tensile force that will act is known and a suitable material with a known value of ultimate tensile strength has been chosen then the cross-sectional area of the rod can be calculated to ensure that the strength of the tie is adequate. The safe working stress used by the designer will be well below the ultimate tensile strength of the chosen material to ensure safety in the event of uncontrollable variables such as flaws in the material or structure or unpredictable variations in loading. The known ultimate tensile strength is generally divided by a **factor of safety**. The value of the factor of safety may lie between 2 and 12, depending upon the nature of the risk involved if a specific type of failure were to occur, e.g. in the design of bridges, aircraft and so forth. A similar concept of factor of safety is also used in discussing how close the normal physiological loading of human tissue structures is to the ultimate strength of the structure, and consequently how efficient the structure is in storing energy.

6.4.2 Viscoelastic materials and strain rate

Viscoelastic structures such as ligaments are of necessity tested in tension to determine their mechanical properties. Because of their time-dependent properties the speed or **rate** of extension is important and must be controlled. The greater the strain rate the greater the stiffness (Figure 6.15(d)).

6.4.3 Example 2

Figure 6.16 shows a tensile stress–strain curve for a ligament, which was elongated at a constant speed. Assuming that the ligament had an effective length of 50 mm and a cross-sectional area of 10 mm² before testing, determine the following:

1. the modulus of elasticity in Pa;
2. the yield stress in Pa;
3. the ultimate strength in Pa;
4. the ultimate strength in N;
5. the maximum elongation before rupture.

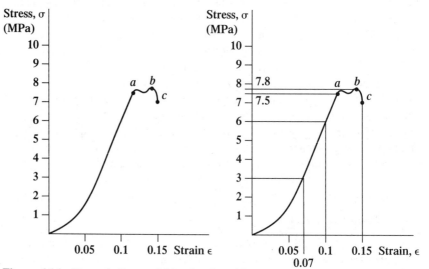

Figure 6.16 Example 2. a = yield point; b = ultimate strength; c = rupture.

Solution:

1. The modulus of elasticity, E

E = the slope of the straight-line portion of Figure 6.16

$$= \frac{\text{change in stress}}{\text{change in strain}}$$

$$= \frac{(6 - 3)}{(0.1 - 0.07)} \times 10^6$$

$$= \frac{3}{0.03} \times 10^6$$

$$= 1 \times 10^8 \text{ Pa.}$$

Note that stress is cited in MPa in Figure 6.16, i.e. 10^6 Pa (or 10^6 N m^{-2}).

2. The yield stress
   Many materials do not possess a well-defined yield point. The best estimate in this case is the **proportional limit**, i.e. the point at which the graph departs from the straight line, which will also coincide with the elastic limit, i.e. point a in Figure 6.16, where $\sigma = 7.5 \times 10^6$ Pa.

3. The ultimate strength in Pa
   By inspection the ultimate strength, point b, is $\sigma = 7.8 \times 10^6$ Pa.

4. The ultimate strength in N

$$\sigma = 7.8 \times 10^6 \text{ Pa (or N m}^{-2})$$

also $\sigma = \dfrac{\text{force}}{\text{area}}$

force = $\sigma \times$ area
$$= 7.8 \times 10^6 \times 10^{-5} \text{ N}$$
$$= 7.8 \times 10 \text{ N.}$$

5. The maximum elongation before rupture
   By inspection, the maximum strain before rupture, $\epsilon = 0.15$.

$$\epsilon = \frac{\Delta L}{L}$$
$$\Delta L = \epsilon \times L$$
$$= 0.15 \times 50$$
$$= 7.5 \text{ mm}$$

6.5 COMPRESSION, STABILITY AND BUCKLING

In structural design terms columns, pillars and struts are elements designed to withstand compressive loads; struts are generally regarded as light structural elements. The mathematical relationships for linear stress, strain and modulus of elasticity that apply to structures under tension also apply to structures in compression. Some materials, such as cast iron, are weak in tension and strong in compression and it is necessary to know whether the material properties,

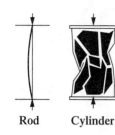

Rod   Cylinder

Figure 6.17 Buckling.

such as ultimate strength, relate to a tensile or a compressive test. Deformation and fracture of the infrastructure will almost certainly depend upon the type of loading that the structure is subjected to.

It is fairly obvious that some structures, such as pulley cords and human ligaments, can only sustain tensile loads; however, regardless of the material used, if any structure is too slender it will be unstable and will **buckle** sideways under compressive forces. Buckling may occur in very slender columns and struts and in thin-walled beams, plates and shells (Figure 6.17).

With respect to the human body, buckling as a particular aspect of the stability of structures is much less important than the fundamental problem of the intrinsic stability of human structures, which includes joints already described in Chapter 3; for example, instability of the lower leg depends upon the tensile properties of the ankle ligaments and the high stresses that result from large moments of force around the ankle joint and not upon any buckling effect that relates to measures of 'slenderness' of the structure.

6.5.1 Degrees of freedom

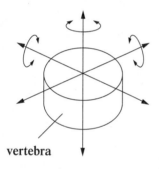

vertebra

Figure 6.18 Six degrees of freedom illustrated on a 'vertebra' from the spine.

A structure that is free to move in space has six **degrees of freedom** with respect to a three-dimensional frame of reference, e.g. translation along and rotation around sagittal, frontal and transverse axes (Figure 6.18). In general the smaller the number of degrees of freedom the more stable the structure.

The shape of a structure obviously affects its freedom of movement. For example, if the socket of an artificial limb or the cuff of an appliance worn by a patient has a circular cross-section that matches that of the limb itself (Figure 6.19(a)), then the socket or cuff will turn more readily during use, tending to shear the underlying soft tissue and causing discomfort or injury to the patient. Relative movement between the structures would be constrained by using a quadrilateral or elliptical cross-section if possible (Figure 6.19(b)).

By examining the degrees of freedom of each structure acting at individual human articulating joints a more analytical approach to the mechanisms of joint stability is possible.

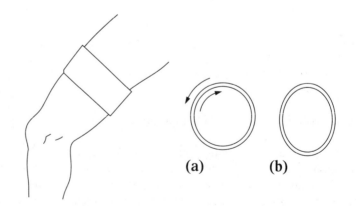

(a)   (b)

Figure 6.19 Structural shape and freedom of movement. (**a**) Relative motion occurs. (**b**) Relative motion is restrained.

6.5.2 Strength, stiffness and shape of structural sections

Experience shows that it is much easier to bend a thin beam than a thick beam, even if the area of the cross-section is identical; simply trying to bend a wooden or plastic ruler will easily confirm this (Figure 6.20(a)).

Formulae for two basic types of simple, linear elastic beams in Figure 6.20(b, c) show that the deflection of a beam under load is inversely proportional to the **cube** of the depth of the beam and that the maximum linear stress that occurs at the outer edges of the beam is inversely proportional to the **square** of the depth of the beam. This means that the effective stiffness and strength of a beam increases considerably as its depth or thickness is increased.

Doubling the depth of a bath seat will make it eight times stiffer. Ribs and corrugations are particularly effective methods of improving the stiffness of a structure to bending loads without adding too much weight (Figure 6.20(d)). Fracture of a beam will tend to start at an outer edge, where maximum fibre stress exists (Figure 6.20(e)), and the type of fracture will relate to the strength of the material in tension, compression and shear.

Formulae for a circular shaft in Figure 6.21 show that, provided the material is only being stressed within the linear elastic range, the angle of twist of a shaft subjected to a torque is inversely proportional to the **fourth power** of the diameter of the shaft and that the maximum shearing stress which occurs at the outer surface of the shaft is inversely proportional to the **cube** of the diameter of the shaft.

6.5.3 Alternative and combined loading modes

The formulae for the deformation of a structure and the stress distribution within a section of a structure that is being bent or twisted take into account the way in which the material is distributed across the section. The influence of the geometrical properties of the cross-section are included in a factor called the **area moment of inertia** in bending and the **polar moment of inertia** in torsion.

Because maximum stresses occur at the outer surfaces of elastic structures that are being bent or twisted, circular or rectangular **tubes** can be quite efficient load-bearing structures. Comparison of the strength and stiffness of a circular tube with a rectangular tube of identical cross-sectional area (Figure 6.22(a)) shows that overall the circular tube is more efficient than the rectangular tube when subjected to the range of loading conditions that can occur – tension, compression, bending and torsion – because, although the rectangular tube may be slightly stiffer and stronger in **bending**, it is much less effective at withstanding **torsion**. The stiffness of tubular sections is dramatically reduced if the section has a discontinuity, such as the introduction of a longitudinal slit, for example (Figure 6.22(b)), because this alters the distribution of stress across the section. In such a case the stiffness may be reduced 100-fold or more. The general problem of non-uniform stress distribution is briefly described later.

The tubular cross-section of long bones is particularly effective because of the variety of loading modes that occur in activities of daily living. As well as being subjected to a variety of loading modes, a long bone such as the femur

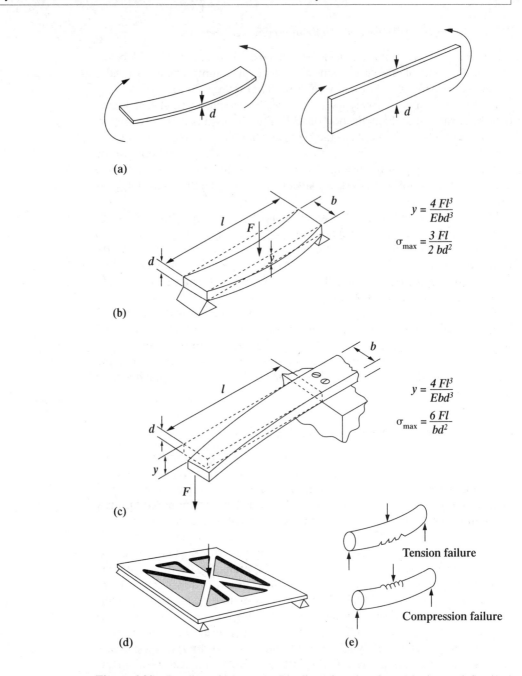

Figure 6.20 Bending of beams. (**a**) Bending of a ruler. (**b, c**) Maximum deflection y and stress (σ_{max}) under load of (**b**) a simply supported beam and (**c**) a cantilever. (**d**) Ribs to improve stiffness of structure. (**e**) Fracture of simply supported beams under load.

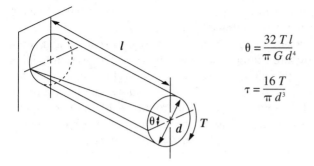

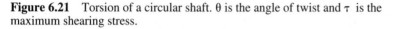

$$\theta = \frac{32\,T\,l}{\pi\,G\,d^4}$$

$$\tau = \frac{16\,T}{\pi\,d^3}$$

Figure 6.21 Torsion of a circular shaft. θ is the angle of twist and τ is the maximum shearing stress.

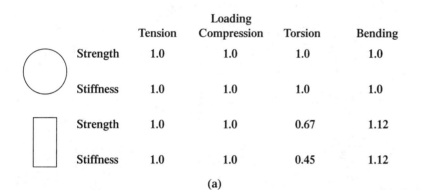

			Loading		
		Tension	Compression	Torsion	Bending
	Strength	1.0	1.0	1.0	1.0
	Stiffness	1.0	1.0	1.0	1.0
	Strength	1.0	1.0	0.67	1.12
	Stiffness	1.0	1.0	0.45	1.12

(a)

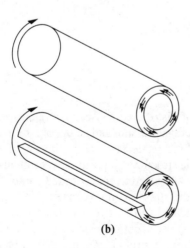

(b)

Figure 6.22 Relative strength and stiffness of tubes. **(a)** Comparison of circular and rectangular tubes. **(b)** Closed and open sections.

is a good example of a structure that can be subjected to combined loading modes, e.g. direct compression combined with bending and/or torsion. In linearly elastic problems where the deformations are small the stress and strain at any point in the structure can be determined by considering each loading mode as though it was acting alone; the stress and strain at that point resulting from the combined loading is then calculated by simple addition or vector addition as required. This approach to solving problems of structures under complex loading modes is referred to as the **method of superposition**. A simple example of stress superposition is illustrated in Figure 6.23.

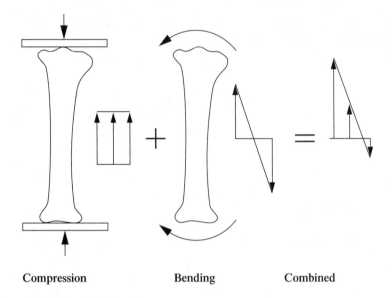

| Compression | Bending | Combined |

Figure 6.23 Combined loading.

6.6   DISTRIBUTED AND CONCENTRATED STRESS

In Chapter 4 the idea of distributed and concentrated forces was introduced together with that of average pressure and actual pressure distribution. A similar concept, only this time related to stress, plays a very important part in understanding why some structures fail. From experimental methods it can be shown that, in a column subjected to concentrated compressive forces F (Figure 6.24(a)), although the stress is approximately uniformly distributed at a mid section of area A and equal to the average stress, $\sigma = F/A$, at sections close to the applied force the stress is not distributed evenly and maximum stresses well in excess of the average stress exist and tend to be concentrated in the region of the concentrated force.

Experimental work also shows that stress concentrations occur at regions in a structure where there is a sudden change of section, such as at sharp corners, at notches, holes and so forth (Figure 6.24(b)). In man-made structures good design involves ensuring smooth and not sudden discontinuities in shape (Figure 6.24(c)).

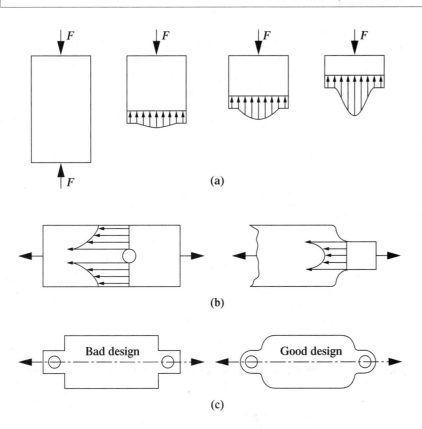

Figure 6.24 Concentrated stress. (**a**) Stress distribution near a concentrated force. (**b**) Stress concentration at discontinuities in structures. (**c**) Good design avoids sharp discontinuities in shape.

6.6.1   Hardness

Surface defects such as scratches also cause stress concentrations and the surfaces of surgical implants such as artificial hips are highly polished to minimize failure originating from surface scratches. **Hardness** is a measure of the resistance of a material to scratching or indentation and it is therefore a mechanical property that is relevant both to the strength of a structure and to its surface wear.

6.7   UNIAXIAL, BIAXIAL AND TRIAXIAL STRESS AND STRAIN

During a simple uniaxial tensile or compressive test, in addition to the linear strain along the longitudinal axis there is a lateral strain along the axis that is perpendicular to the applied force (Figure 6.25(a)).

The relationship between these two perpendicular strains is described by a constant of proportionality called Poisson's ratio (symbol v, nu), i.e. lateral strain $= - v \times$ longitudinal strain. The negative sign indicates that as, say, the 'length' of a section increases when stretched then its 'breadth' decreases and *vice versa*.

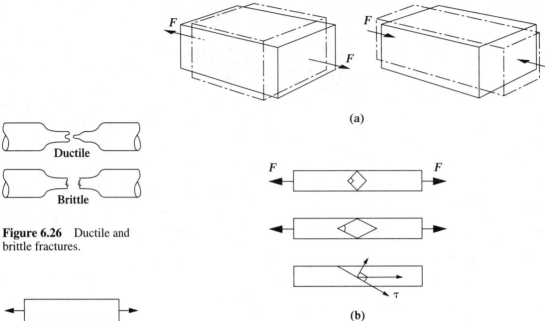

(a)

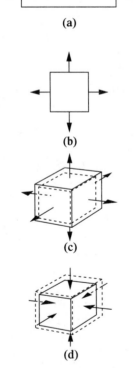

Ductile

Brittle

Figure 6.26 Ductile and brittle fractures.

(a)

Figure 6.25 (**a**) Lateral contraction or expansion associated with an axial force (the Poisson effect). (**b**) Indirect shear stress (τ) arising from direct axial load (F).

(b)

(c)

(d)

Figure 6.27 Uniaxial, biaxial and triaxial loads. (**a**) Uniaxial load (tensile load illustrated). (**b**) Biaxial load. (**c**) Triaxial load. (**d**) Hydrostatic pressure.

It is also apparent from Figure 6.25(b) that by selecting a different plane, one that is inclined to the longitudinal axis, internal equilibrium can be interpreted in terms of shear stress. Shear strain can be seen to be occurring on this plane because by definition shear strain is measured by a change in angle. In practice, ductile materials tend to yield and fail along the planes where shear stresses are maximal and brittle materials tend to fail along planes where direct stresses are maximal (Figure 6.26).

The terms uniaxial, biaxial and triaxial are used in relation to the number of stresses required to completely describe the state of stress in a structure: uniaxial requiring only one stress, e.g. in the case of an axially loaded structure such as a tendon under tension, biaxial for two-dimensional cases, such as skin being stretched along two axes over a flexed muscle; and triaxial for three-dimensional cases (Figure 6.27 a–c). A special case of triaxial stress arises when a body is subjected to a uniform fluid pressure on all sides, which is referred to as **hydrostatic** compressive stress. The ratio of the hydrostatic compressive stress to the decrease in volume of the body is a type of elastic modulus called the **bulk modulus** (Figure 6.27(d)).

Complex loading of a structure may well involve biaxial or triaxial stresses and strains but in the main the properties of materials are determined from simple axial tensile tests. Consequently, alternative theories of failure have been proposed that relate the more complex loading to simple axial tensile test results. The concept of a **principal** stress is relevant to these theories where a principal stress is a direct tensile or compressive stress acting on a plane on which there is **no shear stress**. The **maximum principal stress theory** proposes that failure will occur when a principal stress reaches the yield point of the material as measured in a simple uniaxial tensile test. The **maximum shear stress theory** proposes that failure will occur when a shearing stress reaches the value of the shearing stress that occurs at yielding in a simple uniaxial tensile test.

Reference was made earlier to **membrane stresses** in thin shells. The relationship between pressure, tension and curvature derived to analyse thin shells can be useful in understanding the forces generated by strapping and by other patient supports where a thin flexible material conforms to the curvatures of the body. This will now be examined before dealing with the final topic in this chapter – dynamic stress and strain.

6.8 CIRCUMFERENTIAL TENSION, MEMBRANE STRESS AND STRAPPING

It is intuitively obvious that the 'tighter' a sling or strap is pulled around a part of the body the greater will be the interface pressure on the body at the area of contact, i.e. as the tension in the fabric increases, the pressure at the fabric–body interface increases. It is less obvious how the curvature of the interface affects the relationship between pressure and tension. In fact, for a given tension in the fabric, the greater the radius of curvature the smaller the interface pressure, or in other words the 'flatter' the surface the smaller the pressure. Note that a perfectly flat surface has an **infinite** radius of curvature.

As an analogy, consider what happens when a soap bubble is blown: as the pressure in the bubble increases by blowing, the soap film is stretched, increasing the tension in the film, but as the bubble expands the radius of curvature also increases and it becomes correspondingly easier and easier to blow up the bubble.

Two radii may be needed to describe the curvature of a surface at a particular point. For example, a 10 cm diameter cylinder has a 5 cm radius of curvature in one direction and an infinite radius of curvature in another direction (i.e. it is **flat** along the axis of the cylinder).

The sheet of fabric shown in Figure 6.28 has a radius of curvature R_1 when viewed in the direction B indicated and a radius of curvature R_2 when viewed at a right angle to this direction, in direction C. The tension T, which is the force per unit width at the edge of the fabric, may also be different in these two directions. The equation that relates the pressure, P (i.e. force per unit area on the surface of the fabric), the tension, T, and the radius of curvature, R, is:

$$P = \frac{T_1}{R_1} + \frac{T_2}{R_2}$$

If one of the radii of curvature, say R_2, is infinite, i.e. the sheet is flat in one direction, then

$$\frac{T_2}{R_2} = \frac{T_2}{\infty} = 0 \text{ and } P = \frac{T_1}{R_1}.$$

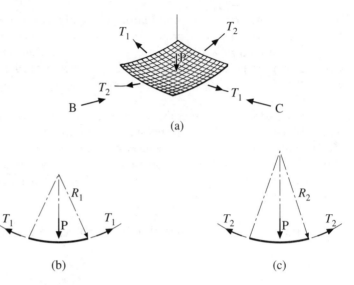

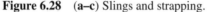

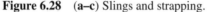

(a)

(b)   (c)

Figure 6.28 (a–c) Slings and strapping.

To take a simple example, if a strap supporting the back of the patient is stretched with a uniform 'tension' around the body, then, because the radius of curvature at the sides of the body is about one-third that at the back of the trunk, the pressure against the skin at the sides of the body would be about three times that which is acting over the flatter region of the back (Figure 6.29).

Similarly, if a hoist sling under the buttocks and thighs had a uniform tension throughout, then areas such as the ischial tuberosities, where the radii of curvature are small, would be subjected to higher pressures than surrounding areas where the radii of curvature are large. Bearing in mind that sling fabrics transmit tensile forces, if it is desirable to redirect or redistribute forces, e.g. to give a more acceptable support pressure pattern, then rigid supports can be incorporated into the sling arrangements (Figure 6.30).

These rigid structures will carry the necessary compression, shear, bending and torsion forces in addition to tension forces.

The above relationships can be expressed in terms of tensile stresses, σ_1 and σ_2, by including the thickness of the 'membrane', t.

$$\frac{P}{t} = \frac{\sigma_1}{R_1} + \frac{\sigma_2}{R_2}$$

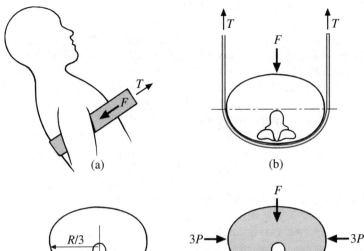
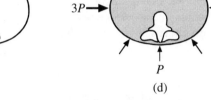

Figure 6.29 (**a–d**) The effect of curvature.

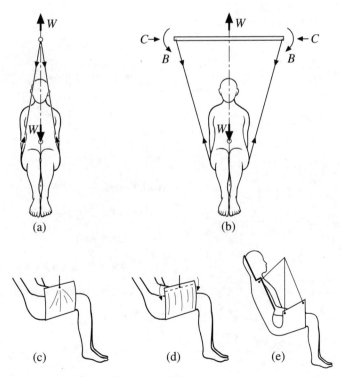

Figure 6.30 (**a–e**) Redistribution of forces.

6.9 STATIC AND DYNAMIC LOADS

A dynamic load infers that the dimension of **time** must be included in the analysis. Generally speaking, three alternative methods of analysing dynamic problems are available (Chapter 7), all based on Newton's second law, force equals mass times acceleration, in one form or another. Broadly, these three methods are (1) the **force–acceleration method**, (2) the **work–energy method** and (3) the **impulse–momentum method**.

The methods of static analysis can be applied to a body that is accelerating uniformly by applying a principle, known as the **d'Alembert principle**. The force required to accelerate the part in question is calculated using Newton's second law, force = mass × acceleration. By applying this force to the centre of mass of the part in a direction **opposite** to the acceleration the dynamic problem is reduced to one of statics (Figure 6.31).

Where this approach is unsatisfactory, e.g. where impact loading or fluctuating loading occurs, the work–energy approach is most commonly used; the concept of **strain energy** is important here.

Uniform acceleration, a

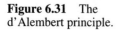

mass, m

Force required for equilibrium
$F (= - m \times a)$

Figure 6.31 The d'Alembert principle.

6.9.1 Strain energy

When a force moves through a distance in the direction of the force it does work. Stress multiplied by its respective area is an internal force and if this pro-

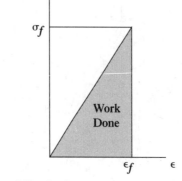

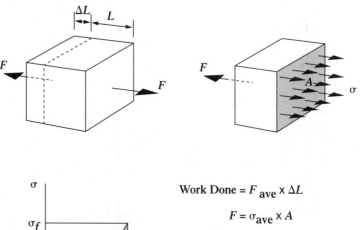

Work Done = $F_{ave} \times \Delta L$

$F = \sigma_{ave} \times A$

$\Delta L = \epsilon \times L$

Work = $\sigma_{ave} \times A \times \epsilon \times L$

$A \times L = 1$ (unit of volume)

$\therefore$ Work = $\sigma_{ave} \times \epsilon_f$

$$= \frac{\sigma_f \times \epsilon_f}{2}$$

Figure 6.32 Strain energy.

duct is multiplied by deformation then this is a measure of the internal work done in a body. For a small unit cube of material under tension the deformation can be related to the linear strain multiplied by its respective initial length. Where stress and strain are increasing linearly from 0 to final values of σ_f and ϵ_f, the work done is computed from the average force and consequently the average stress that acted during deformation. The average stress in this case equals half the final stress. The result is that the work done in a body is related to the product of stress and strain divided by 2 (Figure 6.32). As energy is defined as the capacity of a body to do work, $(\sigma_f \times \epsilon_f)/2$ is a measure of the elastic strain energy per unit volume of the material and is equivalent to the area under the stress–strain diagram (Figure 6.32). An analogous argument can be applied in the case of shearing stresses.

Within the elastic limit the strain energy is stored and hence recoverable. Beyond this point the strain energy is absorbed by the plastic deformation of the structure (Figure 6.33).

The ability of a tissue to either store and return energy like an elastic band or to absorb and dissipate energy like a lump of plasticine naturally affects its role in the body. These properties also affect the type of fracture that results from traumatic injuries. For example, when an extended elastic band snaps the stored energy is suddenly released, with dramatic effect. Because of the viscoelastic nature of tissue the strain rate (or the rate of loading) affects the stress–strain curve and consequently the strain energy that is stored and that which is absorbed (Figure 6.34).

It can be shown that when a bone is loaded rapidly to fracture it behaves differently from the case of slow loading; in the former case the stored strain energy is suddenly released at fracture, causing splintering and further damage to surrounding soft tissues.

Using strain energy concepts it is shown in Chapter 7 that if a load that is held just above the surface of an elastic body is suddenly released the impact causes a maximum deformation twice that achieved by applying the same load slowly. Consequently the maximum dynamic strain and the maximum dynamic stress are twice that of the static case. Under these conditions the body would oscillate and finally come to rest with a deformation and internal stress equal to that which would result from a static load (Figure 6.35).

It is important to note that this doubling of the stress results from a load that is released from just above the surface of the body; dynamic conditions can lead to stresses well in excess of this and in engineering design empirical data is essential in allowing for impact stresses. Conversely, failure of a structure can also result from stresses that are **less** than the ultimate strength of the material if the structure is subjected to repetitive loading; this is called **fatigue** failure (Figure 6.36).

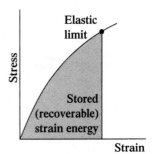

Figure 6.33 Stored and absorbed strain energy.

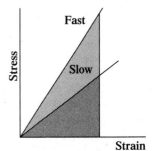

Figure 6.34 Strain energy, viscoelasticity and strain rate.

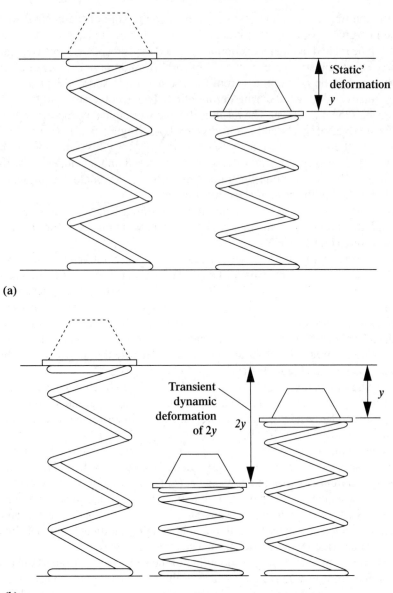

Figure 6.35 Dynamic *versus* static loading. (**a**) Slow application of load. (**b**) Sudden application of load.

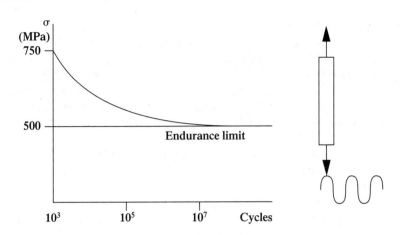

Figure 6.36 Fatigue failure.

6.10 VISCOELASTICITY: CREEP AND STRESS RELAXATION

Strictly speaking as viscoelastic materials exhibit time-dependent behaviour, i.e. they tend to **flow** with time, the stresses and strains associated with loads on such materials are dynamic. The branch of physical sciences that deals specifically with the flow of materials is called **rheology**. In this science conceptual models have been proposed to examine two basic rheological properties; elasticity and viscosity (Figure 6.37). For the linearly elastic spring (Figure 6.37(a)), stress is proportional to strain. For the dashpot containing viscous liquid (Figure 6.37(b)), stress is proportional to strain **rate**.

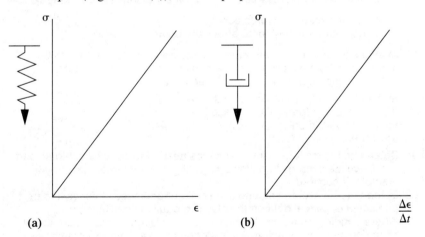

Figure 6.37 Viscoelastic models: springs and dashpots. (**a**) Linearly elastic spring. (**b**) Viscous dashpot.

The three-element model shown in Figure 6.38(a), which is used in biomechanics to examine the behaviour of collagenous tissue, is a very simplified model but it serves to illustrate the two important phenomena of creep and stress relaxation.

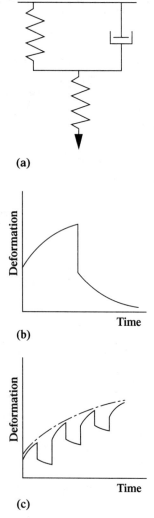

(a)

(b)

(c)

Figure 6.38 Creep.
(a) Three-element model.
(b) Creep. (c) Repetitive
loading.

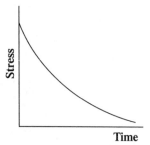

Figure 6.39 Stress
relaxation.

With regard to creep, when a load is applied to this combined model there is an immediate elastic deformation of the bottom spring followed by a slow creep as the deformation of the upper spring is retarded and controlled by the viscous dashpot. On removal of the load there is an immediate recovery of the bottom spring to its original length followed by a delayed recovery of the upper spring, again controlled by the viscous element (Figure 6.38(b)). Repetitive loading will lead to cumulative creep (Figure 6.38(c)).

Stress relaxation occurs when following the loading of the model the overall deformation is held constant. The load required to hold this fixed deformation is reduced with time as the upper and lower springs accommodate to each other with time (Figure 6.39).

The stability of human joints depends upon the integrity of the ligamentous tissue, sustained loading will cause creep and fixed deformation will be accompanied by stress relaxation of these tissues.

6.11 SUMMARY

The basic steps involved in analysing the stresses and strains in a structure are summarized in Figure 6.40. Most of the theories on stress analysis of structures assume that loads are applied within the **linear** range of the material's stress–strain behaviour.

1. Prepare a free body diagram
   (a) Isolate the body or the part of the body of interest.
   (b) Indicate all external force vectors acting on the body.
2. Determine reaction forces by applying the conditions for equilibrium:
   i.e. no net (resultant) force acting
         no net moment of force about any point.
3. At a section of the body/structure where stress and/or strain is to be determined isolate a portion of the body to one side of the section. Determine whether or not external loads arise from:
   (a) axial forces (perpendicular to the section);
   (b) shear forces (parallel to the section);
   (c) bending moments;
   (d) torques.
4. Determine the system of internal forces needed to balance external loads and calculate average stresses by dividing these internal forces by the area of the section.
5. Determine the average strains at a section from these stresses and from published empirical data on the elastic moduli of specific materials.
6. Where bending moments, torques or sharp discontinuities in structural shape occur over a section, a knowledge of area moments of inertia, polar moments of inertia and/or empirical data on stress concentration is required to calculate stress or strain at any point on the section as stress distribution over the section will not be uniform. The total stress/strain at any point resulting from combined loading may be determined using the, method of superposition.

Figure 6.40 Introductory steps in stress analysis of a linearly elastic structure subjected to static loading.

The **mechanics of solid deformable bodies** deals with the **internal** effects of **externally** applied forces.

A **structure** is a physical entity of a definite size and shape that usually carries a load, transmits motion or secures other structures in position.

A **homogeneous** material has a uniform **distribution** of the material constituents.

An **isotropic** material has uniform **mechanical** properties in all directions.

Muscle is an **active** tissue in that it can convert chemical energy into mechanical energy to generate force, unlike connective tissue, which is a **passive** tissue.

The main mechanical criteria for an effective structure are adequate **strength**, **stiffness** and **stability**.

Load is the amount of force acting on one side of a section of a structure.

Stress is a technical term used to express the **load per unit area** acting on a given plane within a material.

Tensile and compressive stresses, σ, are known as **normal** stresses, i.e. they act normal or perpendicular to a given plane.

$$\sigma = \frac{\text{Load (N)}}{\text{Area (m}^2)}$$

Shear stress, τ, acts **parallel** to a given plane.

$$\tau = \frac{\text{Load (N)}}{\text{Area (m}^2)}$$

Strain is a technical term used to express the **deformation** of a body as a ratio of the original dimensions of the body.

Tensile and compressive strains, ϵ, are **linear** strains.

$$\epsilon = \frac{\text{change in length } (\Delta L)}{\text{original length } (L)}$$

As linear strain, ϵ, is a ratio of two lengths it has no unit of measurement.

Shear strain, γ, is a measure of the change in angle between two lines drawn on a surface and it is measured in radians.

The relationship between two perpendicular strains is described by a constant of proportionality called **Poisson's Ratio** (symbol ν, nu), i.e.:

Lateral strain = $-\nu \times$ longitudinal strain

A **principal stress** is a direct tensile or compressive stress acting on a plane on which there is no shear stress.

The **maximum principal stress theory** proposes that failure will occur when a principal stress reaches the yield point of the material as measured in a simple uniaxial tensile test.

The **maximum shear stress theory** proposes that failure will occur when a shearing stress reaches the value of the shearing stress that occurs at yielding in a simple uniaxial tensile test.

The **modulus of elasticity** (**Young's modulus**) for linear stress and strain is

$$E = \frac{\sigma}{\epsilon} \text{ N m}^{-2} \text{ or Pa}$$

A **tangent modulus of elasticity** may be used where a non-linear elastic response exists for any portion of the curve that approximates linearity.

The **shearing modulus of elasticity (the modulus of rigidity)** is

$$G = \frac{\tau}{\gamma} \text{N m}^{-2} \text{ or Pa}$$

When a body is subjected to a uniform fluid pressure on all sides the stress is referred to as **hydrostatic** compressive stress. The ratio of the hydrostatic compressive stress to the decrease in volume of the body is a type of elastic modulus called the **bulk modulus**.

Bending of structures occurs when forces produce equal and opposite moment actions about a section of a structure. The internal effect of bending on a **beam** is to stretch the outer surface of the beam and to compress the inner surface.

A **cantilever** is a beam that is fixed or supported at one end only.

The **neutral axis** of a beam is a longitudinal axis that is neither stretched nor compressed. In a linearly elastic material the stress increases linearly from zero at the neutral axis to a maximum at each edge. In cases where beams are subjected to vertical shearing forces there is also a horizontal shear stress acting along the neutral axis.

Torsion of a structure occurs because of the moment action of a force about the **longitudinal axis** of a structure such as a shaft. In this case shearing stresses act on planes which are **perpendicular** to the longitudinal axis. In a circular cross-section shaft of linearly elastic material maximum shear stress acts at the outer edge of the shaft.

A **membrane** is an element that can be used to analyse thin, shell-like structures such as hollow, thin-walled cylinders or spheres, or strapping and fabric slings.

The equation that relates the pressure, P, (i.e. force per unit area on the surface of the membrane), the tensile stresses, σ_1 and σ_2, the thickness of the membrane, t, and the radii of curvature, R_1 and R_2, is:

$$\frac{P}{t} = \frac{\sigma_1}{R_1} + \frac{\sigma_2}{R_2}.$$

Elasticity is a property of a material that describes its ability to return to its original size and shape immediately after a deforming force is removed. In an elastic material stress is a function of strain.

Plasticity is a property of a material that describes its ability to remain permanently deformed after a deforming force is removed.

Viscoelasticity is a property of a material that describes its time-dependent elastic behaviour. In a viscoelastic material stress is a function of strain and strain rate.

Creep is the **deformation** that continues to occur in a viscoelastic material under a constant load.

Stress relaxation is the **reduction in stress** that occurs in a viscoelastic material under constant deformation.

If the stress–strain graph for a material is a straight line the material is said to obey **Hooke's law**.

The **elastic limit** of a stress–strain graph is that point beyond which full elastic recovery is not possible.

Yield point is that point on a stress-strain graph where yielding of a material begins and plastic deformation occurs. Many materials do not possess a well-defined yield point and the elastic limit is used as an estimate.

In **ductile** materials, i.e. materials that deform extensively before fracture, the yield point is just beyond the elastic limit and deformation increases without any increase in force at this point.

Brittle materials are not capable of withstanding large strains whereas ductile materials are.

The area under a stress–strain curve is a measure of the energy storage and absorption capacity or **toughness** of a material and is closely related to the concepts of ductility and brittleness.

Ultimate tensile strength is the highest stress a material can sustain before fracture.

In design, a working stress is based on the known ultimate tensile strength divided by a **factor of safety**. The value of the factor of safety may lie between 2 and 12.

Buckling is one form of instability of a structure and may occur as a result of compressive forces acting on very slender columns and struts and in thin-walled beams, plates and shells under load.

The **intrinsic stability** of human structures is very dependent on the associated articulating joints.

A structure that is free to move in space has six **degrees of freedom** with respect to a three-dimensional frame of reference. In general the smaller the number of degrees of freedom the more stable the structure.

The influence of the geometrical properties of the cross-section of a structure are included in a factor called the **area moment of inertia** in bending and the **polar moment of inertia** in torsion.

Formulae for two basic types of simple, linear elastic beam show that the deflection of a beam under load is inversely proportional to the **cube** of the depth of the beam and that the maximum linear stress that occurs at the outer edges of the beam is inversely proportional to the **square** of the depth of the beam.

Formulae for a circular shaft show that, provided the material is only being stressed within the linear elastic range, the angle of twist of a shaft subjected to a torque is inversely proportional to the **fourth power** of the diameter of the shaft and that the maximum shearing stress that occurs at the outer surface of the shaft is inversely proportional to the **cube** of the diameter of the shaft.

Because maximum stresses occur at the outer surfaces of elastic structures that are being bent or twisted, circular or rectangular **tubes** can be quite efficient load-bearing structures. The stiffness of tubular sections is dramatically reduced if the section has a discontinuity such as the introduction of a longitudinal slit. The tubular cross-section of long bones is particularly effective because it can resist a variety of loading modes.

In linearly elastic problems where the deformations are small the resulting stress and strain at any point in the structure can be determined by the **method of superposition**, where each loading mode is analysed separately and the resultant stress and strain at that point from the combined loading is then calculated by arithmetical or vector addition as required.

Stress concentrations occur at regions in a structure where there is a sudden change of section, such as at sharp corners, at notches and at holes; good design involves ensuring smooth and not sudden discontinuities in shape.

Hardness is a measure of the resistance of a material to scratching or indentation.

The methods of static analysis can be applied to a body that is accelerating uniformly by applying the **d'Alembert principle** where the force required to accelerate the part in question is applied to the centre of mass of the part, in a direction opposite to the acceleration.

Where **impact loading** or **fluctuating loading** occurs the **work–strain energy** approach is used.

If a load that is held just above the surface of an elastic body is suddenly released the impact causes a maximum deformation **twice** that achieved by applying the same load slowly. Consequently the maximum dynamic strain and the maximum dynamic stress are twice that of the static case.

6.12   TUTORIAL PROBLEMS

1. What is the difference between the following terms?
   (a) force
   (b) load
   (c) stress
2. Briefly explain the distinction between the terms **stress** and **strain** when used in biomechanics.
3. (a) What is meant by the term **tangent modulus of elasticity**?
   (b) Why is the concept of tangent modulus particularly applicable to the analysis of the properties of human tissues?
4. What biomechanical role does cancellous bone, under the ends of long bones, play with respect to joints?
5. Tendons must be relatively inextensible but flexible to function near joints. What structural feature facilitates these two properties?
6. Compression between two elastic bodies can also result in disruptive tensile stress; explain.
7. What role does fluid flow play in the biomechanical response of articular cartilage to load?
8. In a normal tensile stress–strain diagram for ligament what is the clinical significance of the **yield point**?
9. During treatment aimed at stretching the connective tissues surrounding a joint, forces applied to the tissues will be more effective if applied slowly; explain.
10. The shape and orientation of a structure's cross-section is as important as the size of the area of the cross-section in resisting deformation under load; explain.
11. Why are the hardness and surface finish of an artificial hip joint important?

Motion and change of motion: introduction to dynamics

7

CHAPTER OVERVIEW

Dynamics is the study of motion (**kinematics**) and the relationship between force and change of motion (**kinetics**). Dynamics, particularly the dynamics of angular motion, can be very daunting because of the complex-looking terms and equations that tend to be generated but, because the human body depends upon rotating limbs for movement, these terms and some basic equations are relevant. In this chapter the basic concepts in kinematics of **displacement**, **velocity** and **acceleration** in relation to **rectilinear** and **curvilinear translation** and **rotation**, which are required to describe any type of motion, are introduced. Angular motion involves the concepts of centripetal acceleration and the associated centripetal and centrifugal forces, which are introduced here. The concepts of work, energy and power, also discussed in Chapter 5, underpin three methods by which Newton's laws of motion are used to solve kinetic problems: (1) the **force–acceleration method**; (2) the **work–energy method**; and (3) the **impulse–momentum method**; these are outlined with the use of simple examples from remedial therapy.

KEY WORDS

- Dynamics, kinematics, kinetics
- Translation, rotation
- Rectilinear translation, curvilinear translation
- Displacement, velocity, acceleration
- Inertia, moment of inertia
- Centripetal force
- Work, energy
- Momentum, impulse

7.1 INTRODUCTION: WHY DYNAMICS?

In Chapter 1 the rhetorical question was posed: 'Which of the following incidents would cause most pain and injury: gently placing a one kilogram block of cast iron on to your foot or dropping the block on to your foot from a height of, say, 1 m?' As we have all experienced knocks and falls at one time or another in our lives we can accept the general notion that dynamic forces in the form of impacts can be traumatic. However our personal experience is simply not adequate for a proper understanding of the true significance of dynamic forces compared to static forces and we need a more systematic approach to this topic.

In the above example if the height through which the block is dropped is reduced to an infinitely small distance (approaching zero) above the foot, and for simplicity the foot is regarded as being comparable to a linearly elastic body, calculation of the peak force that occurs will show it to be **twice** the value of the weight of the block. The kinetic approach that is most useful in analysing this particular problem is the work–energy relationship.

The somewhat surprising proposal that there is a twofold increase in the peak force generated by a mass under the action of gravity by simply dropping it when it is just above an elastic surface instead of slowly placing it on the surface is explained in more detail in section 7.4.6. However, it is important to stress that forces well in excess of twice the apparent static load can occur in other dynamic situations. For example, if a patient under traction was being transported in a bed over a rough surface or over an obstacle such as a threshold between hospital wards, say, the impulsive forces transmitted through the traction system to the patient could be several times the apparent static load being applied in traction (Figure 7.1).

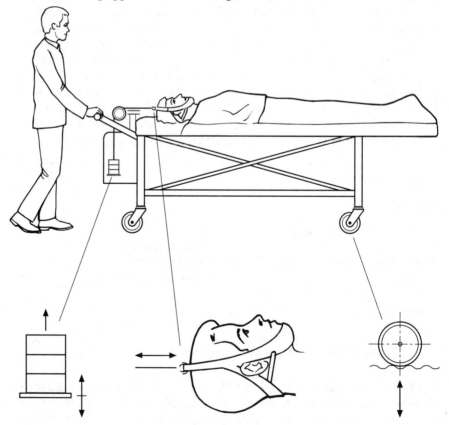

Figure 7.1   Generation and transmission of dynamic forces.

Dynamic forces can of course also assist therapists and patients. Just as a force is required to stop motion one is also required to start motion. Exponents of the martial arts appreciate that it requires less force to redirect a moving body than to stop it. The methods required to safely lift and move heavy bodies should be based on knowledge of fundamental mechanics, particularly the idea of impulse-momentum.

A patient with weak muscles may have difficulty in initiating the movement of a limb but given appropriate assistance to overcome the inertia of the limb he may have little difficulty in completing the motion. Therapists may also use a practical knowledge of basic kinetics to good effect to minimize the forces required to lift and transfer patients. The principles of force and acceleration, impulse and momentum and work and energy, the topics of kinetics, underlie many aspects of clinical practice.

Reference was made above to the work–energy approach to kinetic analysis. Three methods which are used to solve kinetic problems, the force–acceleration method, the work–energy method and the impulse–momentum method, all based on Newton's laws of motion, are discussed later in this chapter; however, it will be useful to introduce ideas related to angular motion first, and the most common type of angular motion is motion in a circle.

7.2 PULLING IN A CIRCLE

At the ice rink some youngsters have been known to form a human chain, holding hands as they circle the rink and, in effect, **rotating** the chain at an ever increasing speed, illustrated schematically in Figure 7.2(a). Even if you have never experienced this personally, you can still visualize the effect. The 'link' youth at the centre of the chain would in effect turn on the spot (the axis) whereas the youngsters at the ends of the chain would travel fastest, i.e. in terms of the speed around the arc of the circle of motion, or the **tangential** speed. In terms of **angular** speed (or velocity) everyone is travelling at the same rate, analogous to the hands of a clock sweeping the same **angle** of rotation each second. In fact if each person in the chain did **not** cover the same angle of sweep in unison then the chain would not stay in a straight line. As we will see later in the chapter the tangential speed increases as the distance from the axis, r, increases, even if the angular velocity is the same for everyone.

Youngster **B** in the chain has to hold on to the outer person, youngster **A**, with an inward pulling action. The **inward** pulling force is called **centripetal** force. But, for every action force there is an equal and opposite reaction force (Newton's third law): **A** pulls on **B** with an equal and opposite force. The **outward** pulling force is called **centrifugal** force.

If **B** lets go of **A**, **A** will not move outward along the line of the chain. Instead, s/he will move in a straight line at a tangent to the arc of motion at the instantaneous linear speed s/he had at the point of loss of grip (Figure 7.2(b)). This is in keeping with Newton's first law, i.e. that a body in motion will continue to move at a constant speed in a straight line unless an external force acts. The centripetal force was the external force, acting to pull the body inward and continuously changing its direction so that it moved in a circular path. Even if the speed of the body around the circular path is constant, because its direction is changing from that of a straight line, its velocity is changing because velocity is a vector quantity and by definition it is accelerating. This inward acceleration is called **centripetal acceleration**.

It is important to systematically examine motion and change of motion and that unfortunately leads to the introduction of some equations. Equations *per se*, are commonplace in engineering analysis, but are much less commonly used in remedial therapy practice. In the following sections the most common equations of motion are presented to highlight the similarities and important differences in describing linear and angular motion.

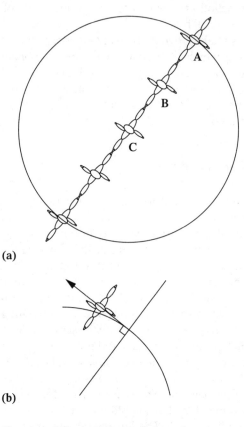

(a)

(b)

Figure 7.2   (**a, b**) Centripetal force: a human chain on ice.

7.3   MOTION AND CHANGE OF MOTION

In statics we deal with stationary bodies or bodies that we can treat as though they were stationary. In dynamics we analyse motion and the forces that are required to initiate, to change and to stop motion.

7.4 KINEMATICS

Kinematics, which can be described as the geometry of motion, is part of dynamic analysis. In remedial therapy, motion analysis of patients, how they move their limbs, walk, get in and out of chairs and so forth, is a major part of practice, and judgements on what constitutes normal and abnormal motion require some form of statement from the observer. Kinematics provides a quantification and precision to these statements. For example, in examining the pathological gaits of patients while it is still useful to identify characteristic **limps** it is proving more useful to use the systematic methods developed in kinematics. Parameters such as length, displacement, angle and time can be estimated or measured and recorded. Observations are made on each body segment or joint (trunk, pelvis, hip, knee, ankle and foot) in addition to the body as a whole. Measurement of the patient's walking speed can be used as an indication of his or her progress in rehabilitation. This approach not only contributes to rationalizing the diagnosis of the origin of locomotor problems but also makes the comparison of treatment regimes and the recording of the progress of patients more universal and more reliable than that based solely on the subjective and personal experience of skilled therapists. The fundamental parameters to be studied are angular and linear **displacement**, **velocity** and **acceleration**.

By restricting our discussion to what is referred to as **plane motion**, i.e. motion in a single plane, the basic parameters of kinematics can be covered without the added difficulty of introducing three dimensional geometry. Plane motion can be fully described in terms of (1) **rectilinear translation**, (2) **curvilinear translation** and (3) **rotation**. Figures 7.3 and 7.4 illustrate the essential difference between each of these three terms.

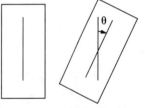

Figure 7.3   Rotation.

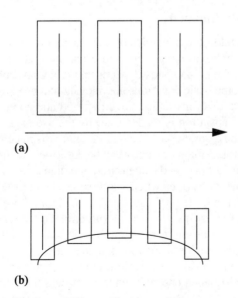

(a)

(b)

Figure 7.4   (**a**) Rectilinear and (**b**) curvilinear translation.

In plane motion **rotation** involves a change in angle of any straight line drawn on the plane of the body with respect to the reference axes of the plane (Figure 7.3. In the rotation of a rigid body all particles in the body, except those lying along the **axis of rotation**, move in a circular path about the axis. The axis of rotation may be permanently at rest, as in the case of a fixed axis or it may be considered to be instantaneously at rest. The idea of an instantaneous axis or **instantaneous centre of rotation** is important in analysing the motion of human joints such as the knee joint.

In **translation** a straight line drawn on the body will remain parallel when the body moves whether the motion is in a straight line, i.e. rectilinear translation (Figure 7.4(a)), or following a curved path, i.e. curvilinear translation (Figure 7.4(b)).

Plane motion can therefore be fully described by a combination of translation and rotation (Figure 7.5).

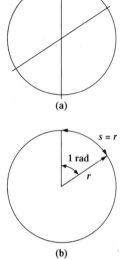

(a)

(b)

(c)

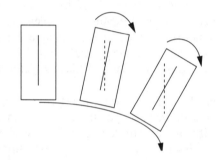

Figure 7.5 Plane motion: translation and rotation.

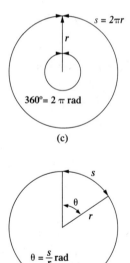

(d)

Figure 7.6 The radian. (**a**) Angular displacement. (**b**) One radian (1 rad). (**c**) $360° = 2\pi$ rad. (**d**) $\theta = s/r$ rad.

7.4.1 A way with equations

Dynamics, particularly the dynamics of angular motion, can be very daunting because of the complex-looking terms and equations that tend to be generated. However, because the human body depends upon rotating limbs for movement, these terms and some basic equations are relevant and need to be introduced.

Kinematic equations for rotation are simplified and comparison with similar equations for translation is made easier by the use of the **radian** (symbol rad), rather than the degree as a measure of angular displacement (Figure 7.6).

The angular displacement of a body can be described by the motion of a line on the body (Figure 7.6(a)), and is measured in radians, where one radian is the angular displacement traversed when a compass, say, set to a radius r, inscribes an arc of circumferential length also equal to r (Figure 7.6(b)). If we used the compass, still set to a radius r, to draw a full circle, the circumference would, by definition of the constant π, measure $2\pi r$ (Figure 7.6(c)). If an arc of circumferential length r encloses one radian then an arc of circumferential length $2r$ encloses 2 radians and an arc of circumferential length $2\pi r$ encloses 2π radians. The angular displacement required to inscribe a full circle also measures $360°$, hence:

2π radians $= 360°$
and as π $= 3.1416$
then 2π $= 6.283$
$\therefore$ 1 radian $= \dfrac{360}{6.283}$
$= 57.3°$

If the compass is set to a radius r and inscribes an arc of circumferential length s, then the enclosed angle $\theta = s/r$ radians (Figure 7.6(d)).

Angular velocity (symbol omega, ω) is defined as the rate of change of angular displacement (symbol theta, θ) (Figure 7.7(a)):

$$\omega = \frac{\text{displacement (radians)}}{\text{time (seconds)}}$$

$$= \frac{\theta}{t} \text{ rad s}^{-1}.$$

Angular acceleration (symbol alpha, α) is defined as the rate of change of angular velocity, ω (Figure 7.7(b)):

$$\alpha = \frac{\text{change in angular velocity (rad s}^{-1})}{\text{time (s)}}$$

$$= \frac{\omega_f - \omega_i}{t} \text{ rad s}^{-2},$$

where $\omega_f - \omega_i$ is the change in angular velocity over a time interval, t. The subscripts, i and f, are used to label an initial velocity, ω_i, and a final velocity, ω_f. The most elegant notation for describing and developing the equations of motion are those used in mathematical **calculus**, which allows the analysis of

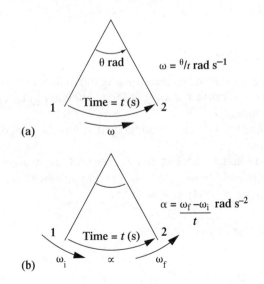

Figure 7.7 Angular velocity and acceleration. (**a**) Average angular velocity, ω. (**b**) Angular acceleration, α.

the motion of a body or particle in relation to the concept of **finite** motion as the sum of **infinitely small** changes in displacement, velocity or acceleration occurring over infinitely small time intervals.

7.4.2 Average angular velocity and constant angular acceleration

Angular velocity is said to be **constant** if equal angular displacements are traversed in equal time intervals. If the velocity is changing then the **average velocity**, ω, over a specified time or over a specified displacement can be computed by dividing the total specified displacement by the total time required to traverse that displacement, i.e.:

$$\omega = \frac{\theta_{total}}{t_{total}}$$

If the velocity is changing at a constant rate, in other words if the angular acceleration, α, is constant, then the average velocity, ω, of, say, ω_i and ω_f is half their sum.

$$\omega = \frac{\omega_i + \omega_f}{2}$$

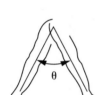

(a)

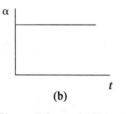

(b)

Figure 7.8 (a, b) Example 1: angular motion of a limb.

(a) Example 1

With reference to Figure 7.8(a), a limb swings through an angle of 0.5 rad (approximately 30°) in 0.2 s. If the limb is initially at rest and the angular acceleration is constant, find:

1. the value of the angular velocity of the limb after 0.2 s;
2. the value of the constant angular acceleration of the limb during this part of the swing.

Solution:

List the known data:

- The initial velocity, αI, is zero because the limb is initially at rest.
- The total displacement, θ, over the time interval of interest is 0.5 rad.
- The total time, t, is 0.2 s.
- The average velocity can be found by dividing the total displacement by the total time.
- Because the angular acceleration is **constant**, the average velocity, ω, can also be computed from the sum of the initial velocity ω_i, which is known (zero), and the velocity ω_f after 0.2 s.

1.

$$\omega = \frac{\theta}{t}$$

$$= \frac{0.5 \text{ (rad)}}{0.2 \text{ (s)}}$$

$$= 2.5 \text{ rad s}^{-1} \tag{1}$$

Also $\omega = \dfrac{\omega_i + \omega_f}{2}$

$= \dfrac{0 + \omega_f}{2}$ $\hspace{4cm}$ (2)

Substituting $\omega = 2.5$ rad s^{-1} from (1) and rearranging equation (2) gives:

$\omega_f = 2\omega$

$\therefore \omega_f = 5$ rad s^{-1}.

Therefore the value of the angular velocity of the limb after 0.2 s is 5 rad s^{-1}.

2.

$\alpha = \dfrac{\omega_f - \omega_i}{t}$

$= \dfrac{5 - 0}{0.2}$

$= 25$ rad s^{-2}

Therefore the value of the constant angular acceleration of the limb during this part of the swing is 25 rad s^{-2}.

7.4.3 Graphs of displacement, velocity and acceleration

Graphs are often used to present kinematic data and in the above example the relationship between angular displacement, velocity and acceleration should become clear if you compare the three graphs in Figure 7.8(b). In each case time is represented on the horizontal axis and displacement, velocity and acceleration are represented on a vertical axis. Over the 0.2 s time interval, displacement increases at an increasing rate (top graph in Figure 7.8(b)), velocity increases in the form of a sloped straight line (middle graph in Figure 7.8(b)) and acceleration, which is constant, is represented as a horizontal straight line (bottom graph in Figure 7.8(b)). If the velocity graph was other than a sloped straight line the calculation of average velocity that involves adding ω_i and ω_f and dividing by 2 would not be valid. Dividing the total displacement, θ, by the total time, t, to find the average velocity, ω, i.e. $\omega = \theta/t$, is, however, valid in all cases.

In the case of motion of a body where acceleration is **constant**, the basic definitions of displacement, velocity, average velocity and acceleration can be algebraically manipulated to derive a set of useful formulae. These are used in Example 4 and are listed in Figure 7.20. Using the formulae it can be shown that, because the acceleration is constant in this case the displacement, θ, is proportional to t^2 in Figure 7.8(b).

7.4.4 Tangential and centripetal acceleration

Tangential acceleration (symbol a_t), is acceleration along the tangent to the path, and centripetal acceleration (symbol a_n) is acceleration normal or perpendicular to the path; centripetal means tending towards the centre. At any point in a rotating body both tangential and centripetal acceleration increase with the radial distance, r, from the axis of rotation of the body (Figure 7.9(a)). The instantaneous velocity, v, of a rotating particle is always tangential to the path of motion (Figure 7.9(b)).

Tangential acceleration, a_t, of the particle arises when the **magnitude** of the tangential velocity changes (Figure 7.9(c)) and it can be shown that $a_t = r \times \alpha$.

Centripetal acceleration, a_n, of the particle arises simply from the change in **direction** of the particle as it follows a curved path (Figure 7.9(d)), and it can be shown that $a_n = r \times \omega^2$.

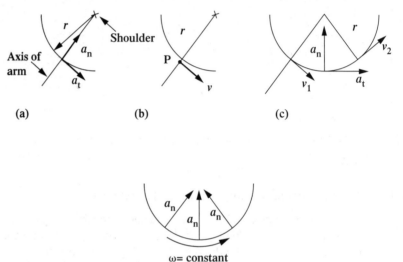

(a)   (b)   (c)

(d)

Figure 7.9 Arm swinging from the shoulder: tangential and centripetal velocity and acceleration. (**a**) a_n and a_t increase as r increases. (**b**) Instantaneous velocity v at point P. (**c**) $a_t = r\alpha$ where $a = (v_2 - v_1)/t$. (**d**) If $\alpha = 0$, i.e. $v_2 = v_1$, then $a_n = r\omega^2$.

7.4.5 Translation

In the translation of a rigid body the paths of all particles of the body are the same and at any instant in time the displacement, velocity and acceleration of all particles are the same. Rectilinear translation, i.e. motion in a straight line, is illustrated in Figure 7.10.

Linear displacement (symbol S) is measured in metres (m), linear velocity (symbol v) is defined as the rate of change of linear displacement and is measured in metres per second (m s^{-1}) (Figure 7.10(a)) and linear acceleration (symbol a) is defined as the rate of change of linear velocity and is measured in metres per second squared (m s^{-2}) (Figure 7.10(b)).

Relationships similar to those proposed above for angular motion can also be stated for linear motion. In other words, linear velocity is **constant** if equal linear displacements are traversed in equal time intervals. If the velocity is changing then the average velocity, v, over a specified time or displacement can be computed by dividing the total displacement by the total time taken to cover that displacement, i.e.:

$$v = \frac{S}{t}$$

If the acceleration, a, is constant, then the average velocity, v, of v_i and v_f is half their sum.

$$v = \frac{v_i + v_f}{2}$$

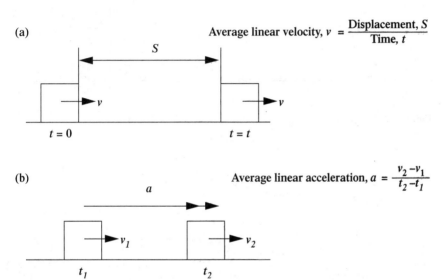

(a)

S

Average linear velocity, $v = \dfrac{\text{Displacement, } S}{\text{Time, } t}$

v

v

$t = 0$ $t = t$

(b)

a

Average linear acceleration, $a = \dfrac{v_2 - v_1}{t_2 - t_1}$

v_1

v_2

t_1 t_2

Figure 7.10   (a, b) Linear velocity and acceleration.

(a) Example 2

With reference to Figure 7.11, a patient in a wheelchair is pushed through a displacement of 1 m in 2 s. If the chair is initially at rest and the acceleration is constant, find

1. the velocity of the chair after 2 s; and
2. the necessary constant acceleration to achieve this velocity.

Solution:
List the known data.

- The initial velocity, v_i, is zero because the wheelchair is initially at rest.
- The total displacement, S, over the time interval of interest is 1 m.
- The total time, t, is 2 s.
- The average velocity, v, can be found by dividing the total displacement, S, by the total time, t.

Because the acceleration is constant the average velocity can also be computed from the sum of the initial velocity, v_i, which is known (zero) and the 'final' velocity, v_f, after 2 s.

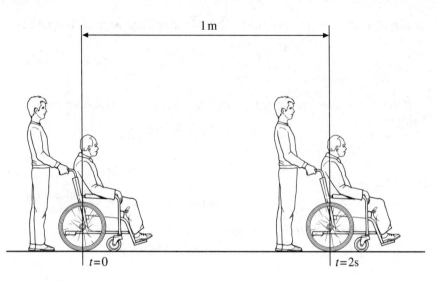

Figure 7.11 Example 2: linear motion – pushing a wheelchair.

(i)
$$v = \frac{S}{t}$$

$$= \frac{1}{2}$$

$$= 0.5 \text{ m s}^{-1} \tag{1}$$

Also $v = \frac{v_i + v_f}{2}$

$$\therefore v = \frac{0 + v_f}{2} \tag{2}$$

Substituting $v = 0.5$ m s^{-1} from (1) and rearranging equation (2) gives

$$v_f = 2 v$$
$$= 1 \text{ m s}^{-1}$$

Therefore the velocity of the chair after 2 s is 1 m s^{-1}.

(ii)
$$a = \frac{v_f - v_i}{t}$$

$$= \frac{1 - 0}{2}$$

$$= 0.5 \text{ m s}^{-2}$$

Therefore the necessary constant acceleration to achieve a velocity of one metre per second in a two second interval is 0.5 m s^{-2}.

7.4.6 Describing complex movements

In Example 2 above, if we examined the motion of the **attendant** rather than the patient then we would see that he does not 'glide' along the path of motion; in other words his body certainly does **not** undergo **rectilinear** translation. His trunk traces a curved path without rotation of any line drawn on it, i.e. it undergoes **curvilinear** translation (Figure 7.12(a)).

His lower limbs undergo both translation and rotation (Figure 7.12(b)); this complex motion can be more simply described by considering the motion at any instant to be the **sum** of a translation and a rotation.

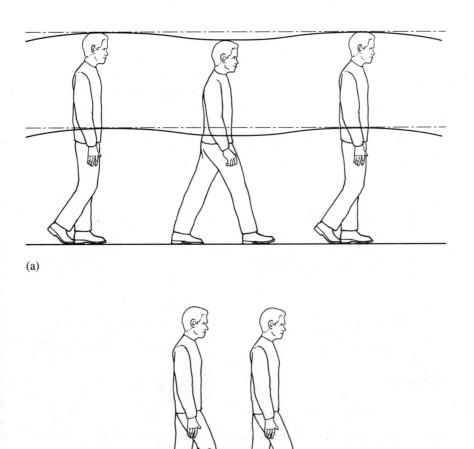

(a)

(b)

Figure 7.12 Motion of the attendant during walking in example 2. (a) Curvilinear translation. **(b)** Translation and rotation.

The average linear velocity, v, of the attendant's centre of gravity over a specified time, t, is the resulting displacement, S, divided by t, i.e. $v = S/t$ (Figure 7.13). This is a good example of the **vector** nature of displacement, velocity and acceleration. Thus with respect to Figure 7.13, if the velocity of interest is that of the body's centre of gravity along the corridor, say, then the displacement of interest is the linear distance from point P_1 to P_2 and not the actual length of the curved path.

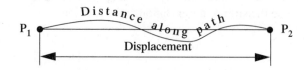

Figure 7.13   The vector nature of velocity.

With respect to the more complex motion of the lower limbs, the velocity, v_A, of any point, A, on the thigh at any instant is the sum of the translation velocity, v_H, of the hip joint, H and the velocity of the point, A, on the thigh relative to the hip joint, $v_{A/H}$. With reference to Figure 7.14, it can be shown that $v_{A/H} = r \times \omega$, where r is the distance of the point A from the axis of rotation, H (i.e. the hip joint) and ω is the angular velocity of the thigh with respect to the hip joint.

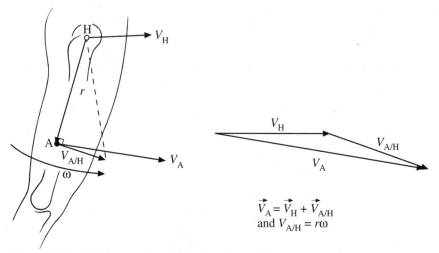

$$\vec{V}_A = \vec{V}_H + \vec{V}_{A/H}$$
$$\text{and } V_{A/H} = r\omega$$

Figure 7.14   Relationship between linear and angular velocity (the arrows above the velocities indicate that velocities are vectors).

7.4.7   Instant centre technique

During motion of the limbs the concept of an instantaneous axis or centre of rotation is used in biomechanical analysis. This is in fact an alternative approach to that of treating a complex motion as the sum of a translation and a rotation. The instant centre technique is best understood graphically (Figure 7.15), and involves finding the point of intersection, O, of the perpendiculars,

R_A and R_B, to the instantaneous velocities, v_A and v_B, at two points, A and B, on the body.

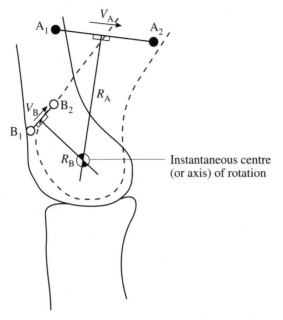

Figure 7.15   Instantaneous centre of rotation.

7.4.8   Relative velocity

Reference was made above to relative velocity. All motions are relative to some frame of reference. Relative velocity is the velocity of an object (or point) A with respect to an object (or point) B. Velocity is a vector quantity and therefore relative velocity must take account of direction as well as magnitude.

Motion of a person on the type of conveyor (moving pavement) found at airport terminals provides a simple example of relative velocity (Figure 7.16). When standing on the conveyor the person's velocity relative to the conveyor is zero while his velocity relative to the wall of the corridor, say, is that of the conveyor, v_c (Figure 7.16(a)). If he is in a hurry and walks with the conveyor with a velocity relative to the moving surface of $v_{m/c}$, then his velocity relative to the wall is now $v_{m/c} + v_c$ (Figure 7.16(b)), whereas if, for some reason best known to himself, he chose to walk against its motion his velocity relative to the wall is now $v_{m/c} - v_c$ (Figure 7.16(c)).

The notation $v_{A/B}$ means the velocity of A with respect to B. Plane motion, treated as the sum of a translation and a rotation, can be effectively described by including this notation (Figure 7.17).

7.4.9   Oscillatory and harmonic motion

If a mass is attached to the end of a spring that is stretched and then released the mass will oscillate to and fro (Figure 7.18(a)). Similarly, if a mass is attached to the end of a length of string to make a simple pendulum (Figure 7.18(b)), which is then displaced and allowed to swing to and fro, the result-

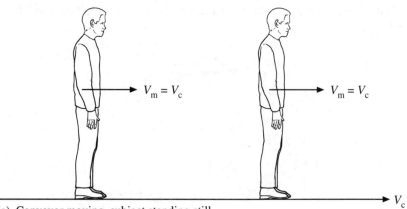

(a) Conveyor moving, subject standing still

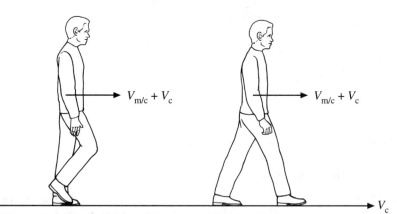

(b) Conveyer moving, subject walking on conveyor

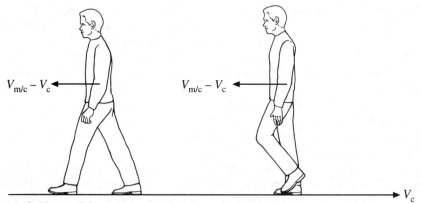

(c) Subject walking in opposite direction to conveyor

Figure 7.16 Relative velocity. (**a**) Conveyor moving, subject standing still. (**b**) Conveyor moving, subject walking on conveyor. (**c**) Subject walking in opposite direction to conveyor.

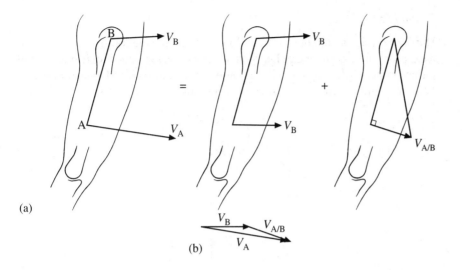

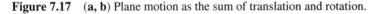

(a)

(b)

Figure 7.17 (**a, b**) Plane motion as the sum of translation and rotation.

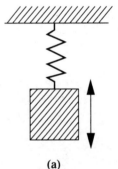

(a)

ing motion has important basic characteristics very similar to what is referred to as **simple harmonic motion**. Mathematical description of oscillatory, harmonic or vibratory motion is somewhat complicated but the relevant parameters of this type of dynamic motion include the concepts of the **amplitude** and **frequency** of the oscillations (Figure 7.18(c)).

7.5 KINETICS

7.5.1 Force, acceleration, mass and centre of mass

Newton's three laws of motion were discussed in some detail in Chapters 2 and 3 and example 3 below is a fairly straightforward example of the application of the force–acceleration method of solving a kinetic problem. Example 4 introduces a slightly more complicated problem. Unlike a simple **rigid** body with a clearly defined centre of mass, the human body is a system of interconnected parts with a less clearly defined centre of mass. Newton's second law, $F = m\,a$, must now be seen as meaning that unless an **external** force acts on a body its **centre of mass** cannot change its state of existing motion. When a swimmer jumps from a diving board, although s/he can twist and turn and in effect change the relative position of the limbs and trunk by muscle action, this has no affect on the trajectory of the centre of mass of the body, which has been determined at the instant that his/her feet lost physical contact with the diving board. Gravity alone now changes trajectory, as it is the only external force acting on his/her body (ignoring air resistance).

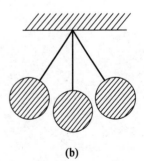

(b)

Figure 7.18 Examples of linear and angular oscillatory motion.
(**a**) Spring mass.
(**b**) Pendulum.

Example 3

During exercise a patient raises and lowers a given weight of mass 5 kg using an appropriate weight and pulley system (Figure 7.19). Ignoring friction in the pulley system what magnitude of force would the patient have to apply to accelerate the weight from rest at a constant rate of, say, 1 m s^{-2}?

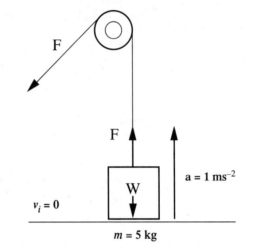

Figure 7.19   Example 3: linear acceleration in a weight and pulley system.

Solution:
With reference to Figure 7.19,

$$W = m\,g$$
where $m = 5$ kg
and $g = 10$ m s^{-2}
Hence $W = 5 \times 10$
$$= 50 \text{ N}$$
$$(F - W) = m\,a$$
$$= 5 \times 1$$
$$= 5 \text{ N}$$
$$F = 5 + W$$
$$= 5 + 50$$
$$= 55 \text{ N.}$$

Note that to simply hold the weight in static equilibrium the patient applies a force equal and opposite to the weight itself (50 N). To raise the weight from rest requires an additional force that is proportional to the acceleration of the weight. In this example a fairly arbitrary nominal value of constant acceleration equal to 1 m s^{-2} has been used and this would require an additional force of 5 N throughout the period of acceleration. In practice, as the pulley is raised against gravity there will be, initially, acceleration to start motion and deceleration as the weight comes to rest at the top of its range of motion. As the weight is then lowered the patient must apply a force **less** than 50 N to control the 'falling' weight. For example, if the patient applies a force of 45 N to the pulley weight then the net **downward** force would now be 5 N (i.e. 50 N − 45 N) and the weight would fall, not with a gravitational acceleration of 10 m s^{-2}, but with a downward acceleration of 1 m s^{-2}.

Example 4: the standing high jump.

This example is based on a very simple practical exercise that the reader can undertake to explore the application of the equations of motion and different kinetic techniques in analysing dynamic forces. With reference to Figure 7.20, if you were to do a standing high jump you would first lower your centre of gravity by flexing hips and knees and then, by rapidly extending the lower limbs, thrust against the floor with an upward force in excess of body weight which accelerates your centre of mass upwards. As your toes leave the floor, your body is fully extended and your 'take-off' velocity is at a maximum. As soon as you lose contact with the floor you can no longer influence the external forces acting on your centre of mass, and gravity, now the only external force acting, slows the body down until it temporarily comes to rest at the maximum height of the jump. You would then 'fall' back to earth and control the force of impact on landing by allowing your hips and knees to flex.

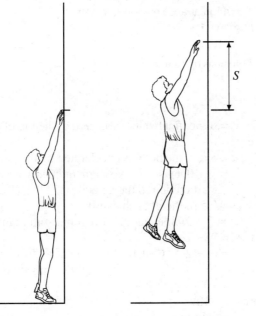

Figure 7.20   Example 4: the standing high jump.

If you estimate the distances that your centre of mass moves at the beginning of the jump, at the point of 'take-off' and at highest point reached during the jump then this information together with your known mass (your body 'weight' in kg) can be used in a variety of dynamic calculations. In practice making chalk marks against a wall with one hand fully extended above the head before and during the jump gives a reasonable approximation to the relevant displacements involved and is something that can be done without any expensive instruments.

1. Calculate the velocity with which you leave the floor if the height reached is 0.5 m using the equation of motion $v_f^2 = v_i^2 + 2a\,S$ (Figure 7.21).

Linear motion	Angular motion
$v_f = v_i + a\,t$	$\omega_f = \omega_i + \alpha\,t$
$v_f^2 = v_i^2 + 2aS$	$\omega_f^2 = \omega_i^2 + 2\alpha\,t$
$S = v_i t + \dfrac{1}{2} at^2$	$\theta = \omega_i + \dfrac{1}{2}\alpha\,t^2$

where
S = linear displacement (m)
v_i = initial linear velocity (m s^{-1})
v_f = final linear velocity (m s^{-1})
a = linear acceleration (m s^{-2})
θ = angular displacement (rad)
ω_i = initial angular velocity (rad s^{-1})
ω_f = final angular velocity (rad s^{-1})
α = angular acceleration (rad s^{-2})
t = time (s)

Figure 7.21   Equations of motion.

$v_f = 0$ (i.e. final velocity is zero at the top of the jump)
therefore $v_f^2 = 0$
$a = g$ (i.e. the body is decelerated by the pull of gravity)
  $= -10$ m s^{-2} ($-$ve sign indicates acceleration opposite direction to the velocity)
$S = 0.5$ m (height achieved)
$v_f^2 = v_i^2 + 2aS$ (equation of motion from Figure 7.21)
therefore $v_i^2 = v_f^2 - 2aS$
  $= 0 - 2 \times (-10) \times 0.5$ (note multiplying two negatives gives a positive result)
  $= 10$
therefore $v_i = \sqrt{10}$
  $= 3.16$ m s^{-1}.

Therefore the velocity with which the body left the floor is just over three metres per second.

2. Calculate the average acceleration and the thrusting force required to achieve the 'take-off' velocity of 3.16 m s^{-1} if the body mass is 50 kg and its centre of mass is raised through a height of 0.2 m during the thrust phase of the jump again using the equation of motion $v_f^2 = v_i^2 + 2aS$ and Newton's second law.

$$v_i = 0 \text{ (i.e. initial velocity is zero at the start of the thrust)}$$
therefore $v_i^2 = 0$
$$v_f = 3.16$$
$$v_f^2 = 10$$
$$S = 0.2 \text{ m (height centre of mass is raised during thrust phase)}$$
$$v_f^2 = v_i^2 + 2\,aS$$

therefore $a = \dfrac{v_f^2 - v_i^2}{2\,S}$ (rearranging the expression to find average acceleration during thrust)

$$a = \frac{10 - 0}{2 \times 0.2}$$
$$= 25 \text{ m s}^{-2}$$

Also $F - W = m\,a$ (i.e. the net force acting on the body)

$$m = 50 \text{ kg}$$
$$a = 25 \text{ m s}^{-2}$$
therefore $F - W = 50 \times 25$
$$F - W = 1250 \text{ N}$$
as $W = m\,g$
$$= 50 \times 10$$
$$= 500 \text{ N}$$
then $F = 1250 + 500$
$$= 1750 \text{ N.}$$

Therefore the average acceleration required in this case is equivalent to 2.5 times the value of the acceleration due to gravity (i.e. 2.5 g) and the thrusting force required is 3.5 times body weight.

7.5.2 Inertia and moment of inertia

Mass is a measure of the quantity of matter that a body contains and the quantity of **inertia** possessed by the body that resists motion, specifically acceleration. **Moment of inertia** is a measure of the resistance that a body offers to **angular** acceleration; it depends upon the mass of the body and the distribution of the mass with respect to the body's axis of rotation.

In the simplest case, if a small mass, m, is accelerating in a circular path of radius r, where the tangential acceleration at any instant is a_t, then the net tangential force, F, causing tangential acceleration is equal to m times a (Newton's second law, $F = m\,a$) (Figure 7.22).

If we now think in terms of **moment of force**, in the above case the moment of force is F times r (force times perpendicular distance to the axis of rotation, in this case the radius of the circle). Consequently, multiplying both sides of the equation $F = m\,a$ by the radius r gives $F\,r = m\,a\,r$ (Figure 7.22).

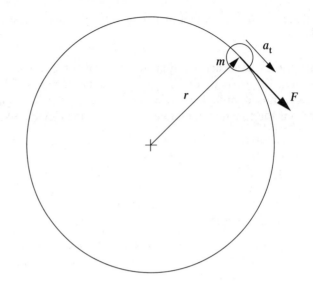

$$F = m \times a_t$$
$$F \times r = m \times a_t \times r$$
$$\text{and } a_t = \alpha \times r$$
$$\therefore F \times r = m \times r^2 \alpha$$
$$m \times r^2 = I$$
$$\therefore Fr = I \alpha$$

Figure 7.22   Moment of inertia (I) for a small mass (m) accelerating in a circular path.

Further, the tangential acceleration, a_t, is equal to the angular acceleration, α, times r ($a_t = \alpha \times r$, see Figure 7.9). Replace a_t by αr in the expression $F r = m a r$, and we obtain $F r = m r^2 \alpha$. For any given body the mass and radius are both constant, which means that the product $m r^2$ is also a constant and it is this constant that is referred to as the moment of inertia and usually given the symbol, I (Figure 7.22).

A mathematical procedure similar to that outlined in Figure 7.22 is used to find the moment of inertia of more complex bodies (Figure 7.23). In effect the body is thought of as composed of an infinitely large number of very small masses each acting at its own radius from the axis of rotation. The sum of all of the individual values of $m r^2$ of these small masses is calculated, using calculus, to determine the overall moment of inertia of the body. In practice, $I = \Sigma m r^2$ (where Σ means 'sum of') becomes $I = M k^2$, where M is the total mass of the body (i.e. Σm) and the distribution of mass with respect to the axis of rotation is described by the **radius of gyration**, k (Figure 7.23).

Example 5

Patients may be encouraged to exercise their limbs over a given range of motion by two different methods: (1) by horizontal movement using a smooth horizontal board to support the limb; and (2) by vertical movement (Figure 7.24). What effect will the weight and size of the limb have in resisting the desired motion in each case?

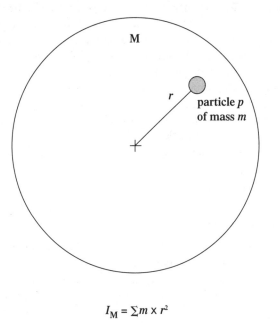

$$I_M = \Sigma m \times r^2$$

Figure 7.23 Moment of inertia for a more complex body.

Solution:
1. In the first case, when the limb is moved over a smooth horizontal board, gravity provides no direct resistance to motion; it could provide indirect resistance in the form of frictional resistance ($f = \mu\, W$) but if the board is smooth this will be minimal. However, during any flexion/extension exercise the fact that the direction of motion is changing means that there is angular acceleration and deceleration occurring. Thus there is some resistance due to the inertia of the mass. In angular motion the moment of force required to cause angular acceleration is related to the moment of inertia ($I = M\, k^2$) and, as the weight of the limb is directly proportional to mass ($W = M\, g$), and the radius of gyration, k, is directly related to the square of the length of the limb, the resistance to motion near the beginning and end of movement is directly related to the weight of the limb and to the square of the length of the limb.

During any part of the motion where the limb is moving at a constant angular velocity there would be no need for a moment of force to overcome inertia ($F\, r = I\, \alpha = 0$, because $\alpha = 0$) but there would be a centripetal force acting throughout directly related to the mass of the limb and the square of the angular velocity ($F_n = m\, r\, \omega^2$). This is the force required to be supplied by the soft tissues around the joint, which will 'pull' on the limb and ensure a circular path of motion (Figure 7.24(a)).

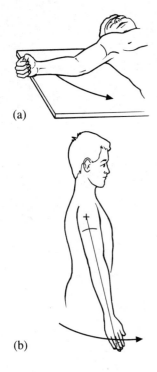

(a)

(b)

Figure 7.24 Example 6: Comparison of motion during exercise in two different gravitational set-ups. (**a**) Horizontal motion of limb on board. (**b**) Vertical motion of limb.

2. In the vertical plane all of the above forces act, i.e. a moment of force is required to accelerate and decelerate the limb, and centripetal force pulls the limb into its circular path of motion. In addition, gravity directly opposes upward motion and assists downward motion (Figure 7.24(b)). The gravitational moment of force arising from the weight of the limb is almost zero when the limb is hanging vertically downwards and increases to a maximum when it is horizontal. Thus the gravitational moment of force increases directly with the weight of the limb and the length of the limb (Figure 7.24(b)). In clinical practice this gravitational moment of force, providing the resistance (during elevation) and the assistance (during depression), will be the dominant force of most interest to the therapist in most cases and its role can be examined by applying the conditions for **static** equilibrium (Chapter 3). Nevertheless, dynamic forces do exist and their significance will increase if the limb is subjected to high speed exercises.

7.5.3 Energy for work

The concepts of work, power and energy were introduced in Chapter 5 in relation to machines. The human body can of course also be viewed in this context, particularly when we are interested in physiological performance during the activities of daily living or during exercise or sport. Again it is important to include angular motion in discussions of work, power and energy when they are applied to motion of the human limbs.

Work

Work is force times displacement in the direction of the force, i.e. Work = $F \times S$ (Figure 7.25(a)). If the displacement is angular displacement, θ, e.g. with respect to lower limb exercise on an isokinetic device (Figure 7.25(b)), then the work can be expressed in terms of $F r \theta$, i.e. the moment of force, $F r$ (or Torque, T) times the angular displacement, θ, which is measured in radians. The unit of work is the **joule**, J (or newton-metre; it is common practice not to include 'rad' in angular units other than angular velocity and angular acceleration).

(b) Power

Power is the rate of doing work, i.e. $F S/t$ or $F v$ (force times velocity; Figure 7.25(a). In angular displacement this becomes $F r \theta/t$ or $F r \omega$ (or $T\omega$) (moment of force or torque times angular velocity; Figure 7.25(b)). The unit of power is the **watt**, W (or joule per second).

(c) Energy

Energy is the capacity of a body to do work, and mechanical energy may take the form of **potential energy** or **kinetic energy** (Figure 7.26(a)). The unit of energy is the same as that of work, the **joule**.

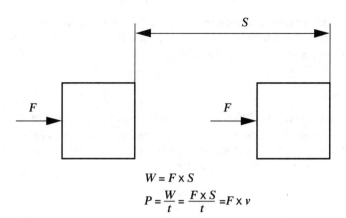

$$W = F \times S$$
$$P = \frac{W}{t} = \frac{F \times S}{t} = F \times v$$

(a)

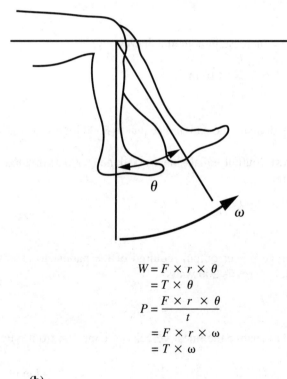

$$W = F \times r \times \theta$$
$$= T \times \theta$$
$$P = \frac{F \times r \times \theta}{t}$$
$$= F \times r \times \omega$$
$$= T \times \omega$$

(b)

Figure 7.25   Mechanical work and power during (**a**) linear and (**b**) angular motion.

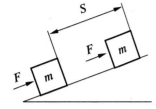

(a)

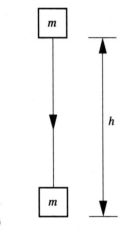

(b)

Figure 7.26 Energy is the capacity to do work and may be (a) kinetic (work = $F \times S$) or (b) potential PE = $m\,g\,h$.

Potential energy is a measure of the work required to raise any mass, m, against gravity to a height, h, above a given reference level point; its value is equal to $m\,g\,h$ (or $W\,h$) (Figure 7.26(b)).

Example 6

A patient who weighs 800 N climbs a flight of stairs in a time of 40 s. If there are 50 steps in the flight and each step is 0.2 m high calculate: (1) the work done by the patient and (2) the average power output required of the patient to achieve this increase in potential energy.

Solution:
1. The total vertical height climbed is equal to the number of steps (50) times the height of each (0.2 m), i.e. 50 × 0.2 m = 10 m.
   The work done by the patient is the work that he does against gravity to increase his potential energy. This is equal to his weight (the vertical force, $W = m\,g$) times the height climbed (vertical displacement, h),

i.e. work done = increase in potential energy
$$= m\,g\,h$$
$$= 800 \text{ N} \times 10 \text{ m}$$
$$= 8000 \text{ J}$$

Therefore the work done by the patient is equal to 8000 joules (8 kJ).

2. The average power output equals the work done (8000 J) divided by the time taken (40 s), i.e.

$$\text{power output} = \frac{8000 \text{ J}}{40 \text{ s}}$$
$$= 200 \text{ W}$$

Therefore the average power output required of the patient to achieve this increase in potential energy is 200 watts.

Kinetic energy

The work required to change the linear velocity of a mass m from v_i to v_f is
$$\frac{m(v_f^2 - v_i^2)}{2}$$
and is equal to the change in the **kinetic energy of translation** $\left[\frac{m\,v^2}{2} \right]$

of the body. Derivation of this expression is presented in Figure 7.27.
   In angular motion the analogous equation for the **kinetic energy of rotation** is

$\left[\dfrac{I\omega^2}{2} \right]$ where I is the moment of inertia of the body and ω is its angular velocity. These relationships are summarized in Figure 7.27.

7.5.4 Conservation of energy

The principle of the **conservation of energy** means that the sum of the potential energy ($m\,g\,h$), the kinetic energy of translation [$1/2\,(m\,v^2)$] and the kinetic energy of rotation [$1/2(I\,\omega^2)$] of a body has a constant value at any time during movement. Any apparent loss in the total mechanical energy calculated at any time would have to be accounted for by the production of energy in another form, such as heat, light or sound.

In Example 6, in practice the patient in climbing stairs will not only have to do mechanical work to increase his potential energy, he will also generate considerable thermal energy in the process. The power **output** is related only to the mechanical work done in increasing his potential energy. The physiological or biochemical power **input** may be some five times this output because the mechanical efficiency of the human body is of the order of some 20% (see Chapter 5 for a discussion on the efficiency of machines). Nevertheless, the principle of the conservation of energy is not violated.

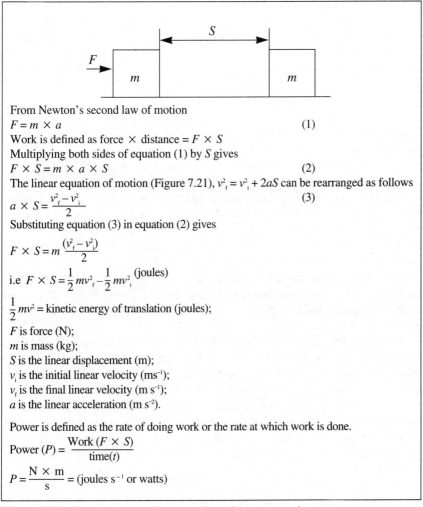

From Newton's second law of motion
$$F = m \times a \tag{1}$$
Work is defined as force $\times$ distance $= F \times S$
Multiplying both sides of equation (1) by S gives
$$F \times S = m \times a \times S \tag{2}$$
The linear equation of motion (Figure 7.21), $v^2_f = v^2_i + 2aS$ can be rearranged as follows
$$a \times S = \frac{v^2_f - v^2_i}{2} \tag{3}$$
Substituting equation (3) in equation (2) gives
$$F \times S = m\,\frac{(v^2_f - v^2_i)}{2}$$
i.e $F \times S = \dfrac{1}{2}mv^2_f - \dfrac{1}{2}mv^2_i$ (joules)

$\dfrac{1}{2}mv^2 =$ kinetic energy of translation (joules);

F is force (N);
m is mass (kg);
S is the linear displacement (m);
v_i is the initial linear velocity (ms^{-1});
v_f is the final linear velocity (m s^{-1});
a is the linear acceleration (m s^{-2}).

Power is defined as the rate of doing work or the rate at which work is done.
$$\text{Power } (P) = \frac{\text{Work } (F \times S)}{\text{time}(t)}$$
$$P = \frac{\text{N} \times \text{m}}{\text{s}} = (\text{joules s}^{-1} \text{ or watts})$$

Figure 7.27 The derivation of the equations for energy and power.

Exercise devices such as treadmills, cycle ergometers and isokinetic machines measure mechanical work and power **output**. Physiological and biochemical measures of, for example, heart rate, respiratory rate, inspired and expired gases, body temperature and blood chemistry are required to estimate the power **input**.

7.5.5 The work–kinetic energy principle

The principle of work and kinetic energy when applied to a body or a system of bodies means that the **sum** of the work of the forces acting upon the body (or system of bodies) equals the change in the kinetic energy of the body (or system of bodies).

In the introduction to this chapter it was said that this principle can be used to show that the peak force arising from releasing a mass m onto the surface of an elastic body, e.g. a spring of stiffness k, is equal to twice the weight, $W = m\,g$, of the mass.

By using the concepts of work and energy we can show that as the height of the mass above the spring, h, is reduced essentially to zero, the **maximum** deflection that the spring experiences before reaching its equilibrium position, ΔL, is in fact equal to $2\Delta L$; consequently the maximum force that occurs during this event is equal to twice k times ΔL, i.e. $2W = 2\,k\,\Delta L$.

Assume that the 'foot', or any other body that the block or mass is dropped on to, is elastic and behaves like a spring with a stiffness k (Nm^{-1}), and that the mass m (kg) has a weight W (N). In a static analysis the mass is 'placed' on the foot and compresses the tissue (the 'spring') until static equilibrium is achieved (Chapter 5); the spring is compressed a distance, ΔL, such that the force provided by the spring, k times ΔL, is equal and opposite to W (Figure 7.28(a)).

In a dynamic analysis the mass is 'dropped' from rest through a small height, h, strikes the top surface of the spring, compresses the spring; overshoots the static equilibrium position, ΔL, because it is still moving at this point, oscillates about this equilibrium position and eventually comes to rest at the static equilibrium position, ΔL (Figure 7.28(b)).

Before static equilibrium is achieved, at the point of maximum spring deflection, ΔL_{max}, the work done by the gravitational force on the falling mass (which by definition, Chapter 5, is assisting the displacement of the mass) is $W(h + \Delta L_{max})$ (Figure 7.28(c)).

The work done **against** the opposing force of the spring is computed from the average force in the spring multiplied by the deformation. For a linearly elastic spring the average force is half the maximum force and hence the work done against the spring is $(F_{max} \times \Delta L_{max})/2$ (Figure 7.28(d)).

The work–energy principle means that the total work of the forces acting on the mass equals the change in the kinetic energy of the mass. However, as the mass is dropped from rest and again comes to rest (temporarily) when the spring is at maximum deformation, the change in kinetic energy is zero (Figure 7.28(c)).

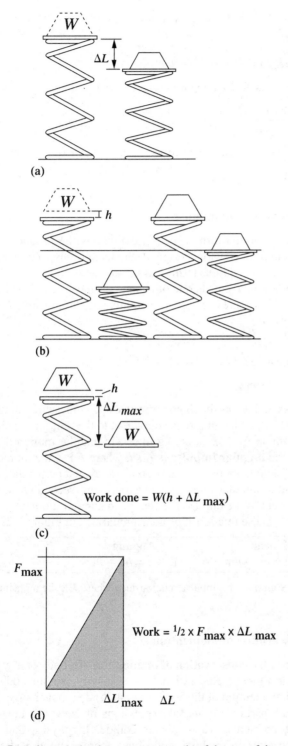

Figure 7.28   Peak force during impact: an example of the use of the work–energy principle. (**a**) Static case. (**b**) Dynamic case. (**c**) Work done. (**d**) Work related to the area under the force–displacement graph.

In this case the work done by gravity equals the work done against the spring giving:

$$W(h + \Delta L_{max}) = \frac{F_{max} \times \Delta L_{max}}{2}.$$

Rearranging the above equation to solve for F_{max} gives:

$$F_{max} = \frac{2W(h + \Delta L_{max})}{\Delta L_{max}}.$$

If $h = 0$, then ΔL_{max} can be cancelled in the above expression, giving:

$$F_{max} = 2W.$$

7.5.6 Momentum and impulse

The concept of **momentum**, which is defined as the product of **mass** and **velocity**, was used in Newton's original statement of his second law. The relationship between the various terms can be seen as follows.

Linear acceleration, a, equals rate of change of linear velocity, $(v_f - v_i)/t$.

Substituting this expression for acceleration into the equation, $F = m\,a$ gives:

$$F = \frac{m(v_f - v_i)}{t}.$$

This expression can be rearranged to give:

$$F\,t = m\,v_f - m\,v_i,$$

where Ft is defined as the **linear impulse** and is measured in units of newton seconds (N s), which in turn is equivalent to the unit for the change in linear momentum, $m\,v_f - m\,v_i$, i.e. kg m s^{-1}. In angular motion the analogous equation for the **angular impulse** is $F\,r\,t$, where $F\,r$ is the moment of force, (or torque, T) acting about some axis on the body at a perpendicular distance, r, and the unit of angular impulse is newton-metre-second (N m s), which in turn is equivalent to the unit for the change in angular momentum, $I\omega_f - I\omega_i$, i.e. kg m^{-2} s^{-1}. These relationships are summarized in Figure 7.29.

Linear	Angular
$F \times t = mv_f - mv_i$	$T \times t = I\omega_f - I\omega_i$

Figure 7.29 Summary of impulse relationships where T is the moment of force or torque.

7.5.7 Conservation of momentum

The principle of the **conservation of momentum** of a body or a system of bodies means that if there are no external forces acting upon the body (or system) then the total momentum of the body (or system) does not change. Impulse and momentum are particularly useful expressions of Newton's laws for dealing with **impact** problems, where bodies collide. In physics and engineering mechanics the concepts of **elastic** collisions, where colliding bodies bounce off each other, and **inelastic** collisions, where bodies stick together after impact, are useful. In biomechanics the impulse–momentum approach is particularly useful for understanding the large impact forces that can arise at human joints during, say, running, or the forces that cause bone fracture during falls. The concept of conservation of angular momentum was briefly introduced in Chapter 1 with respect to the spinning ice skater (Figure 7.30). With arms outstretched the spinning skater has an angular momentum equal to the product of the moment of inertia and angular velocity of the rotating body, i.e. $I\,\omega$ or $m\,k^2\omega$. By drawing arms inwards the skater's radius of gyration, k, is reduced but body mass, m, is unchanged; no external force or moment of force has been introduced, thus the skater's angular velocity must increase to conserve angular momentum, i.e.

$$m\,k^2_{\,1}\,\omega_1 = m\,k^2_{\,2}\,\omega_2$$

$$\therefore \omega_2 = \left(\frac{k_1}{k_2}\right)^2 \omega_1\ .$$

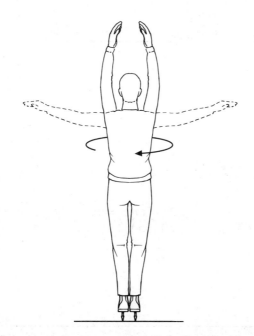

Figure 7.30 Spinning on ice: conservation of angular momentum.

To illustrate the conservation of linear momentum consider two ice skaters, a child (mass m) and an adult (mass $2m$), who are initially at rest, pushing against each other (Figure 7.31). Their respective velocities after the application of this impulsive force will be **inversely** related to their masses, i.e. in this case, the child (mass m) will move twice as fast as the adult ($2m$). Notice that this example highlights the fact that momentum is a vector quantity and the direction (indicated in this case by the minus sign) is important. Note also that the force exerted by the adult on the child is equal and opposite to that exerted by the child on the adult (an illustration of Newton's third law). By using the conservation of momentum we do not have to know the actual values of the force or accelerations involved; the analysis assumes that, when the bodies break contact, forces no longer act and the bodies have reached their respective constant velocities.

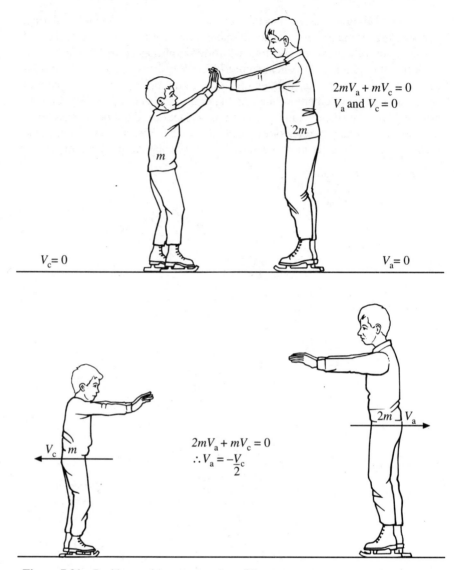

$$2mV_a + mV_c = 0$$
$$V_a \text{ and } V_c = 0$$

$$V_c = 0$$

$$V_a = 0$$

$$2mV_a + mV_c = 0$$
$$\therefore V_a = -\frac{V_c}{2}$$

Figure 7.31 Pushing on ice: conservation of linear momentum.

7.6 SUMMARY

Dynamics is the study of motion (kinematics) and the relationship between force and change of motion (kinetics).

The topics that comprise dynamics are related as in Figure 7.32.

Plane motion can be fully described in terms of (1) **rectilinear translation**, (2) **curvilinear translation** and (3) **rotation**.

An **instantaneous axis** or **centre of rotation** is a point about which a body (e.g. the knee joint) can be considered to be rotating at a given instant in time.

Relative velocity is the velocity of a body or a point on the body with respect to another body or point.

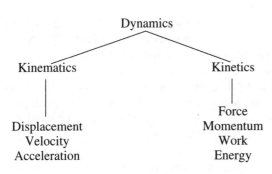

Figure 7.32 Relationship of the topics that comprise dynamics.

Tangential acceleration (symbol a_t) is acceleration of a point along the tangent to a curved path and centripetal acceleration (symbol a_n), is acceleration normal (i.e. perpendicular) to the path. If the point is a distance r from the instantaneous axis of rotation moving with an instantaneous angular velocity ω and an angular acceleration α, then:

$$a_t = r \times \alpha.$$
$$a_n = r \times \omega^2.$$

The following equations of motion can be applied when the acceleration of a body is constant:

Linear motion **Angular motion**

$$v_f = v_i + a\,t \qquad \omega_f = \omega_i + \alpha\,t$$
$$v^2_f = v^2_i + 2a\,S \qquad \omega^2_f = \omega^2_i + 2\alpha\,t$$
$$S = v_i\,t + \frac{1}{2}a\,t^2 \qquad \theta = \omega_i\,t + \frac{1}{2}\alpha\,t^2$$

where
S = linear displacement (m)
v_i = initial linear velocity (m s^{-1})
v_f = final linear velocity (m s^{-1})
a = linear acceleration (m s^{-2})
θ = angular displacement (rad)
ω_i = initial angular velocity (rad s^{-1})
ω_f = final angular velocity (rad s^{-1})
α = angular acceleration (rad s^{-2})
t = time (s).

Three methods by which Newton's laws of motion are used to solve kinetic problems are: (1) the **force–acceleration method**, (2) the **work–energy method** and (3) **the impulse–momentum method.**

Inertia is a measure of the resistance that a body offers to acceleration. Moment of inertia (I) is a measure of the resistance that a body offers to angular acceleration; it depends upon the mass of the body (m) and the distribution of the mass with respect to the body's axis of rotation. The latter is determined by the radius of gyration (k):

$I = m\, k^2$.

Work (unit J) is force times displacement in the direction of the force, i.e. Work = $F \times S$.

Energy (unit J) is the capacity of a body to do work and mechanical energy may take the form of potential energy or kinetic energy.

Power (unit W) is the rate of doing work.

The principle of the **conservation of energy** means that the sum of the potential energy ($m\, g\, h$), the kinetic energy of translation [$1/2(mv^2)$] and the kinetic energy of rotation [$1/2(I\,\omega^2)$] of a body has a constant value at any time during movement. Any apparent loss in the total mechanical energy calculated at any time would have to be accounted for by the production of energy in another form such as heat, light or sound.

Momentum is the product of mass and velocity.

The principle of the **conservation of momentum** of a body or a system of bodies means that if there are no external forces acting upon the body (or system) then the total momentum of the body (or system) does not change.

The following equations are used in kinetic analysis of problems.

	Linear motion	**Angular motion**
Impulse	$F \times t = m\, v_f - m\, v_i$	$T \times t = I\,\omega_f - I\,\omega_i$
Newton's second law	$F = m\, a$	$T = I\,\alpha$
Kinetic energy	$\dfrac{1}{2} m\, v^2$	$\dfrac{1}{2} I\,\omega^2$
Momentum	$m\, v$	$I\,\omega$
Work	$F\, S$	$T\,\theta$
Power	$F\, v$	$T\,\omega$

where
S = linear displacement (m)
v = linear velocity (m s^{-1})
v_i = initial linear velocity (m s^{-1})
v_f = final linear velocity (m s^{-1})
a = linear acceleration (m s^{-1})
θ = angular displacement (rad)
ω = angular velocity (rad s^{-1})
ω_i = initial angular velocity (rad s^{-1})
ω_f = final angular velocity (rad s^{-1})
α = angular acceleration (rad s^{-1})
t = time (s).
m = mass (kg)
F = force (N)
T = torque or moment of force (N m)
I = moment of inertia (kg m^2)

7.7   TUTORIAL PROBLEMS

1. During exercise a patient raises a weight of mass 6 kg through a vertical height of 0.3 m in 2 s. Calculate:
   (a) the work done by the patient; and
   (b) the average power output required of the patient.
2. Calculate the work done in stretching a linearly elastic spring if the maximum force required to stretch the spring by 0.5 m is 40 N.
3. During dynamic muscle performance testing of the extensor muscles of the knee the leg swings through an angle of 0.2 rad (approximately 12°) in 0.2 s. If the leg is initially at rest and the angular acceleration is constant, find:
   (a) the value of the angular velocity of the leg after 0.2 s; and
   (b) the value of the constant angular acceleration of the leg during this part of the motion.
4. Under what conditions could an object continue to travel at constant speed and yet be accelerating?
5. Explain why it is very tiring to walk on a surface such as deep sand.
6. Consider the activity of pushing a heavy patient in a wheelchair. Which aspects of such an activity are likely to prove the most difficult for the attendant?
7. Indicate how each of the following factors determines the extent of injury which may occur due to a fall:
   (a) body mass;
   (b) height of fall;
   (c) compliance of surface of impact.
8. What is the difference between inertia and moment of inertia?

8 A tendency to flow: introduction to fluid mechanics

CHAPTER OVERVIEW

The pressure and the buoyancy that water can provide are used in therapy to treat a variety of problems that patients can have. External fluid pressure applied to a limb can help in the control of oedema. When partially immersed in water in a hydrotherapy pool a patient who has difficulty moving can be assisted by the buoyancy force provided by the water. For the remedial therapist fluid mechanics is relevant in understanding the use of hydrotherapy in patient treatment, mechanisms of human joint lubrication, the behaviour of human connective tissue and the properties of some specific technical aids and equipment used for patient care, e.g. pneumatic splints and water beds. The aim of this chapter is to outline the main principles of **hydrostatics**, i.e. the principles which govern the equilibrium of fluids. The concepts of **viscosity** and **laminar** and **turbulent** fluid **flow** are briefly introduced because of their relevance in understanding the resistance to motion of a **body** in, for example, a hydrotherapy pool and the resistance to motion of a **fluid** (e.g. blood, synovial fluid or air) in a vessel or cavity.

KEY WORDS

- Fluids, liquids, gases
- Adhesion, cohesion
- Viscosity
- Density
- Relative density (specific gravity)
- Pressure
- Pascal's principle
- Hydrostatic pressure
- Buoyancy
- Archimedes' principle
- Centre of buoyancy
- Moment of buoyancy force
- Stability
- Fluid flow
- Poiseuille's law
- Laminar flow, turbulent flow
- Reynold's number

8.1 FLUIDS: LIQUIDS AND GASES

Most solids offer considerable resistance to any force that tends to change their shape. When a shearing force is applied to a solid body it deforms until a new position of equilibrium is reached. In contrast, a liquid or a gaseous 'body' cannot effectively resist any force that tends to shear it and the body deforms continuously, that is, it flows; hence the common term **fluid** (Figure 8.1).

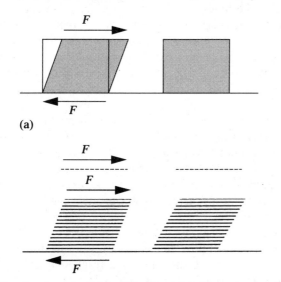

Figure 8.1   The shearing of solids and liquids. **(a)** Solids resist shearing forces. **(b)** Liquids cannot resist shearing: they flow.

The term fluid therefore includes both liquids and gases and a number of mechanical principles can be applied to both states of matter although each also possesses particular characteristics. For example, the volume of liquid in a jar doesn't depend on the shape of the jar, whereas a gas will expand to fill any container. In both cases the mass doesn't change but in the case of the gas the volume does; liquids are virtually incompressible, gases expand and are readily compressed (Figure 8.2).

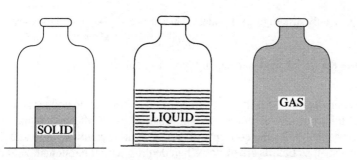

Figure 8.2   Solid, liquid and gas in a 'container'.

The virtual incompressibility of liquids (and solids) can be attributed to a **force of repulsion** that acts between molecules when they are forced very close together. It is however the **force of attraction** that normally exists between molecules that accounts for properties such as surface tension and fluid viscosity. The term **cohesion** is used to describe the attraction between like molecules and the term **adhesion** is used to describe the attraction between unlike molecules. Adhesive forces arising from liquid between the outer surface of the lungs and the inner surface of the chest wall transmit movement of the chest wall to the lungs during breathing. Cohesive forces cause surface tension in fluids within the small mucus-lined sacs called alveoli of the lungs, which contract, expelling gases during breathing.

All real fluids are viscous, i.e. they possess **viscosity**, which is a fluid frictional property that resists shear forces. An **ideal** fluid is assumed to have zero viscosity.

A small element of an ideal fluid may be considered to be similar to a sphere with a frictionless surface to which only forces normal to the surface can be applied. Just as it is not possible to generate a braking force on car wheels on a slippery surface, forces or force components tangential to the surface of the fluid sphere simply cannot be generated (Figure 8.3). It would also be impossible to spin a frictionless sphere, so a fluid element can be visualized as a sliding rather than a rolling element. This image of small frictionless spheres helps to illustrate why water, for example, has to be constrained in a container. The sides of the container provide the necessary normal forces to prevent flow occurring in any horizontal direction as a result of gravity; the base only restrains flow normal to its surface (Figure 8.3).

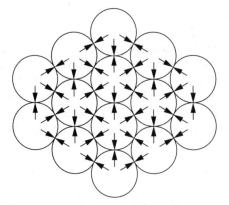

Can only sustain forces normal to the surface

Tangential forces cannot be generated on the surface

Figure 8.3 Ideal fluid element visualized as a smooth sphere.

When dealing with the mechanics of rigid bodies the concepts **mass, force** and **friction** are essential. When dealing with the mechanics of solid deformable bodies the concepts of **stress, strain, elasticity** and structural elements such as **beams** are basic. When dealing with the mechanics of fluids the concepts of **density, pressure** and **viscosity** are fundamental.

8.2 DENSITY

For a given quantity of fluid whose shape can change readily it is much more useful, when it comes to mechanical analysis and calculations, to think of the mass of a small defined unit within the fluid. If we divide the total mass of a quantity of fluid by its total volume then we derive the concept of **mass density** (symbol ρ, rho); in SI units this is expressed in $kg\ m^{-3}$.

$$\text{mass density, } \rho = \frac{\text{mass (kg)}}{\text{volume (m}^3)}$$

If we multiply mass by g, the acceleration due to gravity, then we derive **weight density**.

$$\text{weight density, } \rho \times g = \frac{\text{weight (N)}}{\text{volume (m}^3)}$$

8.2.1 Relative density (specific gravity)

In hydrotherapy it is particularly convenient to use the concept of **relative density**, which is also referred to as **specific gravity** and is the density of a liquid (or solid) relative to that of pure water at its maximum density at 4°C; as this is a ratio it has no units.

Example 1

The density of water at 4°C is $1000\ kg\ m^{-3}$. What is the relative density of ice if its mass density is $920\ kg\ m^{-3}$?

Solution:

$$\text{Relative density of ice} = \frac{920}{1000}$$
$$= 0.92$$

The relative density of a solid body determines whether the body floats or sinks in water. By definition the relative density of water is 1. Matter with a relative density less than 1 will float, e.g. ice floats in water; matter with a relative density greater than 1 will sink (Figure 8.4(a)). In fact the proportion of a floating body under the water is equal to the relative density of the body, e.g. if the relative density of ice is 0.92 then 92% of the volume of the ice will be beneath the surface of the water (Figure 8.4(b)).

The relative density of the human body is of the order of 0.86–0.97; it varies with the amount of air in the lungs during respiration and there is significant variation with age, illness and disability as well as variation between the different tissues of the body. In relation to hydrotherapy the buoyancy and stability of a patient in a pool is dependent on the shape and density of the different parts of the body; this is discussed in section 8.5. First we will consider the important features of **pressure**.

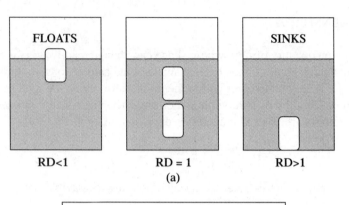

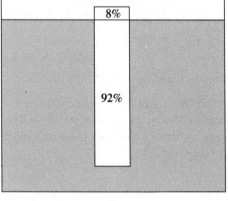

Figure 8.4 **(a, b)** Relative density and flotation.

8.3 PRESSURE

The concept of interface pressure was introduced in Chapter 4, i.e.

$$\text{pressure on a plane surface} = \frac{\text{force acting normal to the surface.}}{\text{area of the surface}}$$

In a fluid, the concept of pressure at a **point** within the body of the fluid is used and this means the normal force that would be applied on a small plane surface of unit area placed at that point; in SI units this is expressed in pascals, i.e. newtons per square metre.

The unit of pressure is named after the 17th-century French philosopher, physicist and mathematician, Blaise Pascal, who is regarded as one of the founders of hydrostatics and hydrodynamics. Pascal proposed the fundamental principle of the transmission of pressure in an enclosed ideal fluid at rest, i.e.

any change in pressure at any point within the confined fluid will be transmitted without loss to all other points of the fluid (Figure 8.5).

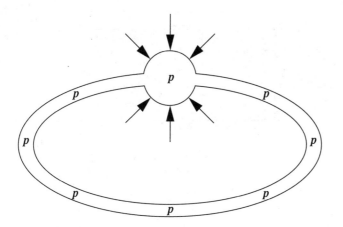

Figure 8.5 Transmission of pressure in a confined fluid: Pascal's principle.

The importance of the property of fluids described by Pascal's principle can be seen in many examples in health care, e.g. in systems that control potentially damaging impulses or high stresses by transmitting and distributing pressure throughout the system, such as fluid-filled mattresses and cushions. Equipment, such as a patient hoist, that uses a hydraulic jack to provide a mechanical advantage illustrates Pascal's principle (Chapter 5).

Pressure can be applied to a fluid externally by a piston or pump. Although the heart is within the body it can also be regarded as applying an 'external' pressure by its pumping action to the enclosed blood within the vascular system. The illustration in Figure 8.5 is deliberately a plan view of a fluid-filled vessel to emphasize that Pascal's principle of pressure transmission is **independent** of gravity. However, the weight of liquid arising from gravity is another source of pressure.

With reference to Figure 8.6(a) it can be shown that the pressure at any particular depth below the free surface of a liquid, caused by the weight of the liquid above, is equal to the vertical distance from the point to the surface multiplied by the weight density of the liquid. Atmospheric pressure due to the weight of the atmosphere above a free surface of liquid would also increase the pressure within the liquid but at this stage we will only consider the distribution of pressure caused by the weight of the liquid itself.

The weight of the column of liquid (Figure 8.6(a)) is equal to the height of the column, h, times the cross-sectional area of the column, A, times the weight density, ρg, of the liquid and this weight must be supported by an upward vertical force acting at the base and equal to the pressure acting at this level, p, multiplied by the cross-sectional area of the column, A. The area A that is common to both sides of the equation cancels out, i.e.

$$p \times A = h \times \rho \times g \times A$$
$$p = h \rho g \text{ (pascals)}$$

This static pressure in a fluid is referred to as **hydrostatic pressure**.

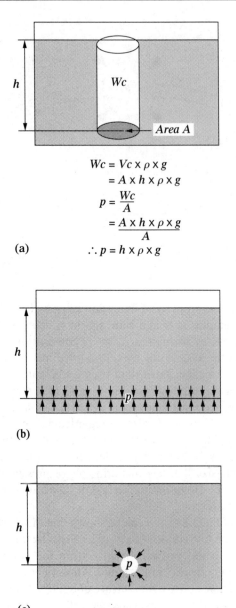

$$Wc = Vc \times \rho \times g$$
$$= A \times h \times \rho \times g$$
$$p = \frac{Wc}{A}$$
$$= \frac{A \times h \times \rho \times g}{A}$$
$$\therefore p = h \times \rho \times g$$

(a)

(b)

(c)

Figure 8.6 (a–c) Hydrostatic pressure.

Although we have used the concept of a column of liquid to determine the pressure at a given level below the free surface, as the area of the column is not included in the final expression for pressure then we can apply this expression to a theoretical 'point' below the surface where the cross-sectional area of the column is infinitely small. In addition, the above argument can be applied to any point on the same horizontal plane (Figure 8.6(b)).

Further, although the above calculation was based on a vertically oriented pressure required to balance the weight of liquid above it, it can be shown experimentally that the same value of pressure would act in all directions at this point (Figure 8.6(c)). This very important property of an ideal fluid arises because of its inability to resist shear forces.

(a) Example 2

With reference to Figure 8.7 an irregularly shaped pool has slanted walls so that the volume of water is difficult to determine. If the depth of the water is 3 m and the mass density of water is 10^3 kg m^{-3}, calculate the hydrostatic pressure at the bottom of the pool.

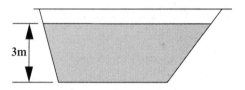
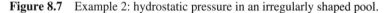

3m

Figure 8.7   Example 2: hydrostatic pressure in an irregularly shaped pool.

Solution:

$p = h \rho g$
$h = 3$ m
$\rho = 10^{-3}$ kg m^{-3}
$g = 9.8$ m s^{-2}

$p = (3$ m$)(10$ kg m$^{-3})(9.8$ m s$^{-2})$
  $= 29\ 400$ N m^{-2}
  $= 29\ 400$ Pa
  $= 29.4$ kPa.

In the above examples we have ignored the additional pressure that the earth's atmosphere exerts near the earth's surface. This additional pressure (which is 1.01×10^5 Pa or 760 mmHg at sea level at 0°C) will be transmitted to **every** point of the liquid (Pascal's principle). When atmospheric pressure is omitted the measured or calculated pressure is referred to as **gauge pressure**. When atmospheric pressure is included the term **absolute pressure** is used, i.e.

Absolute pressure = Gauge pressure + Atmospheric pressure.

In clinical work in particular, pressure is often cited in mmHg (millimetres of mercury) because mercury manometers were commonly used to measure pressure, e.g. blood pressure, for many years. The following example illustrates the relationship between Pa, mmHg and mmH$_2$O.

LLYFRGELL COLEG MENAI LIBRARY
SAFLE FFRIDDOEDD SITE
BANGOR GWYNEDD LL57 2TP

Example 3

If the mass density of water is 10^3 kg m^{-3} and the relative density (specific gravity) of mercury is 13.6, find the hydrostatic pressure at the bottom of a 10 cm column of mercury (Hg) in:
1. mmHg
2. mmH$_2$O
3. Pa.

Solution:
1.

$$p = 10 \text{ cmHg}$$
$$= 100 \text{ mmHg}$$

2.

$$p = h_{water} \times \rho_{water} \times g = h_{mercury} \times \rho_{mercury} \times g$$
$$\therefore h_{water} = h_{mercury} \times \frac{\rho_{mercury}}{\rho_{water}}$$
$$= h_{mercury} \times \text{ relative density of mercury}$$
$$= 100 \times 13.6$$
$$= 1360 \text{ mmH}_2\text{O}$$

3.

$$p = h\,\rho\,g$$
$$= 0.1(\text{m}) \times 13.6 \times 10^3(\text{kg m}^{-3}) \times 9.8(\text{m s}^{-2})$$
$$= 13\,328(\text{kg m s}^{-2})\text{m}^{-2}$$
$$= 13.328 \text{ N m}^{-2}$$
$$= 13\,328 \text{ Pa}$$
$$= 13.3 \text{ kPa}$$

Note that in (3), pressure in pascals was calculated using values of h (in metres) and ρ (density in kg m^{-3}) for mercury but the same answer would have been obtained if equivalent values of these parameters for water had been used, i.e. $h = 1.36$ m and $\rho = 10^3$ kg m^{-3}.

8.3.1   Blood pressure and gravity

Hydrostatic pressure arising from gravity influences blood pressure in different parts of the body and the effect is particularly noticeable in different body positions such as lying, sitting and standing. At this stage the effect can be best understood if we ignore blood flow and think of the circulatory system as a simple closed loop in which the fluid (blood) is at rest. The effect can be compared directly to the analogous 'column of liquid' discussed earlier (Figure 8.8).

Provided the column is sealed at the top to prevent loss, then when in a 'lying' position the pressure is constant along the column; any pressure intensity introduced to the column by, say, a plunger or pump at any point in the system would be transmitted to all other points of the fluid (Pascal's principle; Figure 8.8(a)). In the supine or prone body the pressure in the arteries of the head and feet are approximately equal to that at, and applied by, the heart (Figure 8.8(b)).

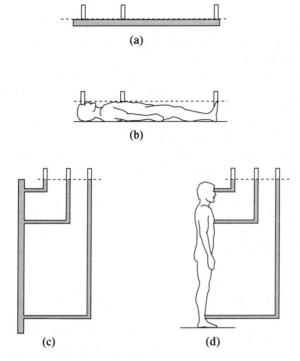

Figure 8.8 (a–d) Blood pressure and gravity.

In the vertical position the hydrostatic pressure due to gravity increases with depth in the column as discussed above (Figure 8.8(c)). In the body in the standing position exactly the same gravitational effects act and although the pressure intensity introduced at the heart must be transmitted without loss to the head and the feet the net result is that the pressure at the head is lower than at heart level and that at the feet is considerably higher (Figure 8.8(d)).

Despite the real complexity of the living circulatory system in contrast to the simple static model used above the influence of gravity on hydrostatic pressure variation can still be appreciated by reference to these basic principles and these are very relevant to the therapist. The increased blood pressure gradient from head to feet can cause oedema (swelling) in the legs. Similarly, in a hydrotherapy pool the water pressure increases with depth and this external pressure on the limb can be used to treat the oedema. During changes in position of the body, e.g. from lying to standing upright, the change in hydrostatic pressure contributes to changes in blood distribution and blood flow in the cardiovascular system. In patients with impaired circulatory systems it is important to ensure that sudden changes in position are avoided because of this influence of gravity on hydrostatic pressure.

While the direct hydrostatic pressure effect of water is in itself valuable there is no doubt that the most important property that water provides in hydrotherapy is **buoyancy**.

8.4 BUOYANCY

When partially immersed in water in a hydrotherapy pool a patient who has difficulty moving can be assisted by the buoyancy force provided by the water. It is important to understand that gravity is still acting directly on the patient's body. The difference is that in the water the body is now also being subjected to upward forces as well, which tend to counter the weight of the immersed limbs and trunk. In fact the buoyancy forces are themselves a result of gravity acting on the water that surrounds the patient. Recall that the pressure increases with the depth below the surface and that a unique property of a fluid is that the pressure at any point in the fluid will be normal to the surface of any body immersed in it. We can visualize this pressure distribution following the contours of the body but increasing in intensity with depth to tend to thrust the body upwards (Figure 8.9(a)).

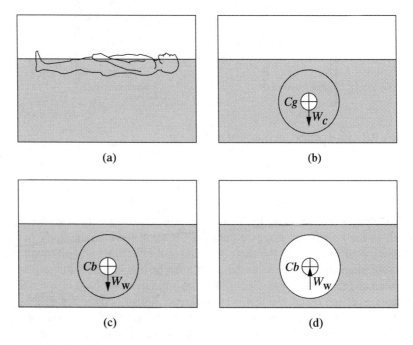

Figure 8.9 **(a–d)** Buoyancy.

To understand how we derive the value of this buoyancy force, again visualize the situation before the body entered the water. For simplicity we will consider a simple shape such as a cylinder rather than the more complex trunk and lower limbs and propose that the cylinder was immersed in the water. The weight of the complete cylinder, W_c, acts at its centre of gravity, Cg, whether on land or in water (Figure 8.9(b)). The space that the cylinder occupied was previously occupied by water (Figure 8.9(c)). This 'block' of water had weight, W_w (equal to its volume times its weight density), and this weight acted downwards at its centre of gravity, Cb (Figure 8.9(c)).

   Despite this downward force the body was in equilibrium. This is only possible if an equal and opposite force is present. The equal and opposite force can only arise from the pressure of the **surrounding** water and the resultant upward force, W_w, must also act at Cb (Figure 8.9(d)). The upward force is the **buoyancy force** and the centre of gravity of the displaced liquid, Cb, is called the **centre of buoyancy**.

   This result is known as **Archimedes' Principle** and can be summarized as follows:

   If a body is wholly or partially immersed in a liquid, it experiences a vertical force (buoyancy force) equal and opposite to the weight of liquid which would occupy the space enclosed by the immersed part of the body (weight of the displaced liquid), and this up-thrust acts through the centre of gravity of the displaced liquid (centre of buoyancy).

   Apart from very sensitive measures of the exact weight of small objects the buoyancy effect of **air** on the weight of a body is negligible. However the buoyancy effect of a liquid such as water on a submerged body is considerable. The term **apparent weight** is used, where:

apparent weight (in water) = actual weight (in air) − buoyancy force

or

buoyancy force = actual weight (in air) − apparent weight (in water).

The buoyancy force is equal to the weight of the displaced water, W_w, which is also equal to the volume of water times its weight density, i.e.

$$\text{buoyancy force} = W_w = V_w \times \rho_w \times g$$
$$\text{and } V_w = \text{volume of the body, } V, \text{ because the body}$$
$$\text{is fully submerged}$$

$$\text{hence buoyancy force} = (\text{volume of the body, } V) \times \rho_w \times g$$

$$= \frac{(\text{weight of body, } W)}{(\text{density of body, } \rho \times g)} \times \rho_w \times g$$

$$= \frac{(\text{weight of body, } W) \times g}{\dfrac{(\text{density of body, } \rho) \times g}{\rho_w}}$$

$$= \frac{\text{weight of body, } W}{\text{relative density of body.}}$$

Example 4

With reference to Figure 8.10, a body is suspended from a spring balance and registers a weight of 8 N. When the body is completely immersed in water the reading of the balance shows 1 N. Find the relative density of the body.

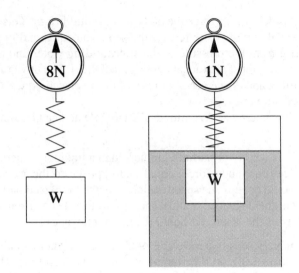

Figure 8.10 Example 4: apparent weight loss of a submerged body.

Solution:

$$\text{Buoyancy force} = \text{actual weight (in air)} - \text{apparent weight (in water)}$$
$$= 8\,\text{N} - 1\,\text{N}$$
$$= 7\,\text{N}$$

$$\text{also, buoyancy force} = \frac{\text{weight of body, } W}{\text{relative density of body}}$$

$$\text{thus, relative density of body} = \frac{\text{weight of body, } W}{\text{buoyancy force}}$$
$$= \frac{8}{7}$$
$$= 1.14$$

The buoyancy force may be referred to as the **apparent weight loss**.

It is very important to realize that the buoyancy force only reduces the apparent weight of the **immersed** part of a body. Thus if a patient is standing in water and the water level is below the hip joints there would of course be no reduction in the gravitational load acting on the hip joints and no buoyancy force acting to unload these joints. The unloading effect at a point on a body, due to buoyancy is related to the level of the point **below** the surface of the water (Figure 8.11).

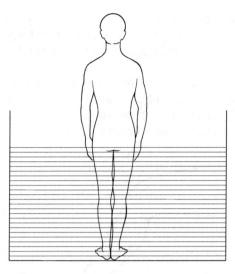

Figure 8.11 Apparent weight loss and a partially immersed body (buoyancy force only reduces the apparent weight of the *immersed* part of the body)

8.5 MOMENTS OF FORCE AND STABILITY

Archimedes' principle is used to advantage in therapy for people with motor difficulties (movement difficulties). If the patient is exercised while partially immersed in water, the buoyancy force aids the patient's muscles. This aid makes greater movement of the extremities possible and helps prevent disuse atrophy. However, the stability of the body in water is different from that on dry land. On dry land stability is related to the position of the body's centre of gravity in relation to its base of support. In water the position of the body's centre of buoyancy in relation to its centre of gravity has the dominant effect on its stability because if the lines of action of body weight and buoyancy force are not coincident, there will be a turning effect on the body (Figure 8.12). Bearing in mind that the centre of buoyancy of an immersed body is

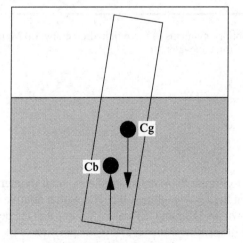

Figure 8.12 Moments of force and stability in water.

equal to the centre of **gravity** of the equivalent volume of water then the centre of buoyancy will lie at the geometrical centre of the body and the centre of gravity will only lie at the geometrical centre when the mass of the body is uniformly distributed.

Weight always acts vertically **downwards** and buoyancy force always acts vertically **upwards**. Consequently, moments of force arising from buoyancy forces acting on limbs that are submerged in water act contrary to moments that arise from the weight of the limb (Figure 8.13).

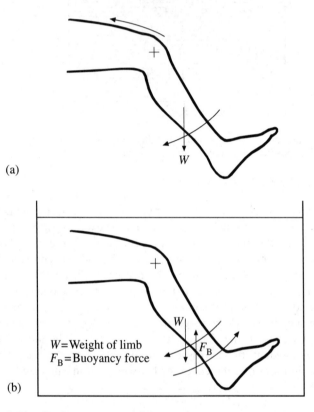

(a)

W=Weight of limb
F_B=Buoyancy force

(b)

Figure 8.13 Contrary moments of force in hydrotherapy. (a) Moment of force in air. (b) Moment of force in water.

Example 5

With reference to Figure 8.14, calculate the external moment of force acting at the knee when the leg, weighing 70 N and with a relative density of 1.1, is extended as shown in (1) air and (2) water. Assume that the position of the centre of buoyancy of the limb coincides with the position of its centre of gravity.

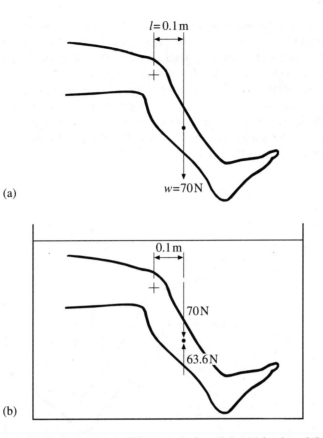

(a)

(b)

Figure 8.14 Example 5: moments of force at the knee joint (a) in air and (b) in water.

Solution:

1. Moment of force at the knee joint = weight of the limb, W × perpendicular distance, l

$$= 70(N) \times 0.1(m)$$
$$= 7 \text{ N m clockwise}$$

2. Buoyancy force, $F_B = \dfrac{\text{weight of the limb}}{\text{relative density}}$

$$= \frac{70}{1.1}$$
$$= 63.6 \text{ N}$$

moment of force at the knee joint $= (W \times l) - (F_B \times l)$
$$= (70 \times 0.1) - (63.6 \times 0.1)$$
$$= 7 - 6.4 \text{ (to nearest decimal place)}$$
$$= 0.6 \text{ N m clockwise.}$$

The external moment of force due to gravity has been essentially eliminated by the counter moment of the buoyancy force. In air, gravity is causing flexion of the knee and the patient would have to resist this external force by the use of knee extensor muscles. If a float, i.e. an object with a very low relative density, was attached to the lower leg (Figure 8.15), then one can see without recourse to calculation that this additional buoyancy force would produce a relatively large counter-clockwise moment of force at the knee joint, i.e. extension of the knee. Thus with such a float the patient would have to use knee **flexors** to resist the external forces in this case.

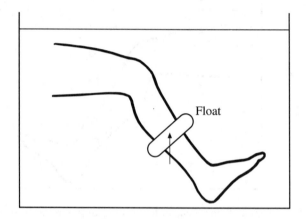

Figure 8.15   Use of floats in hydrotherapy.

8.6   MOVEMENT IN WATER

If a **streamlined** body is moved through water at a slow steady speed a form of friction over the surface of the body causes resistance, which increases as the speed of movement increases (Figure 8.16(a)). If the shape of the body produces what are referred to as eddy currents or **turbulence** downstream in the wake of the body, the resistance is increased by a form of drag and may now be proportional to the **square** of the speed of movement (Figure 8.16(b)). Consequently it is easier to move a body in a pool if the movements are slow and minimize turbulence by, for example cutting through the water with the edge rather than the flat of the hand.

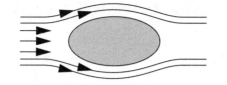

(a)

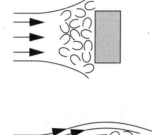

(b)

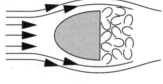

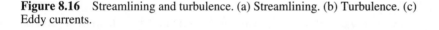

(c)

Figure 8.16 Streamlining and turbulence. (a) Streamlining. (b) Turbulence. (c) Eddy currents.

8.7 FLUID FLOW

Fluid mechanics and particularly fluid dynamics is complex and mathematical models depend extensively on experimental data to ensure valid practical use of any theory. However, flow of any fluid must satisfy the equations of motion, which are still based on Newton's laws, and in addition the concept of **continuity**; the latter basically means that in any closed system there can be no net gain or loss of mass. Thus for an incompressible fluid flowing through a conduit, the volume of fluid (given by the product of the cross-sectional area, A, and the velocity, V, of the fluid) passing through any section must be constant.

The principle of the conservation of energy must also apply to fluid mechanics and in addition to kinetic energy $[(m v^2)/2]$ and potential energy resulting from position in relation to some reference datum $[m g h]$; the concept of **pressure energy** (a form of strain potential energy proportional to the pressure intensity at a given point in the fluid) is used. These concepts are used in engineering to develop equations for the analysis of fluid flow.

Fluid motion in which one fluid layer or **lamina** slides smoothly over another without turbulence is called **laminar** or streamlined flow. Viscous shear in the fluid is the dominant force acting. Water has a fairly low viscosity compared to, say, syrup. Newton's **law of viscosity** relates shear stress and viscosity to the rate of angular deformation of the fluid, which is described in terms of the rate of change of velocity of the fluid normal to the velocity (Figure 8.17), i.e.

$$\tau = \eta \frac{\Delta v}{\Delta y} \text{ (Pa)},$$

where

τ = shear stress

η = viscosity and

$\frac{\Delta v}{\Delta y}$ = rate of change in velocity of the fluid normal to the velocity.

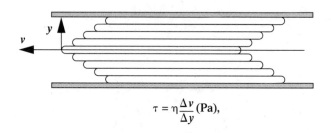

$$\tau = \eta \frac{\Delta v}{\Delta y} \text{ (Pa)},$$

Figure 8.17 Laminar flow: Newton's law of viscosity.

Therefore if a fluid is distorted by, say, the shear stress or the shear forces acting between the surfaces of a synovial joint the resistance to sliding would be expected to vary with the viscosity of the fluid and the rate of distortion on the basis of elementary theory. Of the theories and equations used to analyse fluid flow **Poiseuille's law** is perhaps the most relevant at this level of study to illustrate the implications of this type of analysis to biomechanics.

When liquid is contained in a tube connected to a tank and prevented from flowing by the use of a stopper, measurements of the pressure in the tube will show that (1) the pressure is constant along the length of the tube and (2) the magnitude of this hydrostatic pressure increases with the effective 'head' of liquid (Figure 8.18).

When a liquid flows through the tube there is a pressure drop as energy is used to overcome the resistance of the tube to the flow process (Figure 8.19). The volume of liquid flowing per second, i.e. the flow rate, **increases** as the value of the 'supply' pressure increases relative to the pressure at the exit point of the tube (i.e. the pressure **drop** along the length of tube increases). However the flow rate **decreases** as the resistance to flow increases. This can be summarized as follows:

$$\text{Flow rate} = \frac{\text{pressure drop}}{\text{resistance}}$$

The variables that determine the resistance to flow of an incompressible fluid in a tube when the flow is **laminar**, i.e. streamlined, are related in Poiseuille's law, as follows:

$$\text{Resistance} = \frac{8 \times \text{viscosity of fluid } (\eta) \times \text{length of tube } (l)}{\pi \times \text{radius of tube } (r)^4}$$

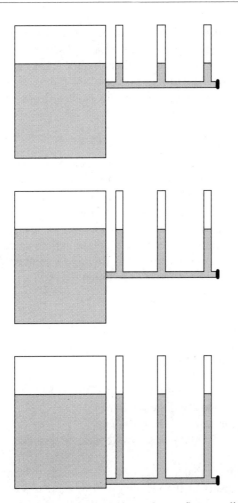

Figure 8.18   Hydrostatic pressure in a tube under no-flow conditions.

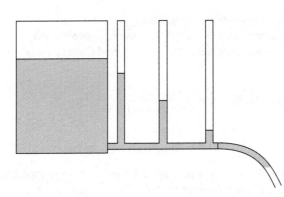

Figure 8.19   Drop in fluid pressure along the length of a tube during flow.

Hence the resistance to flow increases as the **viscosity** (η) of the fluid increases and as the length (l) of the tube increases, which would perhaps follow intuition. However the most dominant factor is the radius (r) of the tube. Resistance decreases as the **fourth power** of the radius. In other words, if the radius of the tube is doubled then the resistance drops by a factor of 16, because:

$$(2r)^4 = 2^4 \times r^4 = 16 \times r^4.$$

Strictly speaking this equation only applies to an ideal fluid undergoing laminar flow but although blood is not an ideal fluid this equation is still useful as a qualitative guide in explaining the important role that vasodilation and vasoconstriction play in controlling blood flow.

Turbulence occurs when fluid swirls and mixes, causing dissipation of mechanical energy, and is related to an increase in fluid velocity past a critical threshold value. An expression known as Reynold's number (R) is used to estimate whether flow will be laminar or turbulent.

$$R = \frac{2\rho vr}{\eta}$$

where ρ = density
v = average velocity
r = radius of tube
η = viscosity of fluid
if $R < 2000$ the flow will be laminar
if $R > 3000$ the flow will be turbulent
if $2000 < R < 3000$ the flow will tend to be unstable.

From this we can see that laminar flow is less likely to be maintained for fluids with a low viscosity as the velocity of flow increases or where the radius of the tube increases. This type of relationship can help to explain the existence of sections of the vascular system where turbulence may occur.

8.9   SUMMARY

The term **fluid** includes both liquids and gases.

All real fluids are viscous, i.e. they possess **viscosity**, which is a fluid frictional property that resists shear forces. An **ideal fluid** is assumed to have zero viscosity:

$$\text{mass density, } \rho = \frac{\text{mass (kg)}}{\text{volume (m}^3)}$$

$$\text{weight density, } \rho \times g = \frac{\text{weight (N)}}{\text{volume (m}^3)}.$$

Relative density, which is also referred to as **specific gravity**, is the density of a liquid (or solid) relative to that of pure water at 4°C. As a ratio it has no units.

In a fluid, the concept of **pressure at a point** within the body of the fluid is used and expressed in **pascals**, i.e. newtons per square metre.

Pascal's principle states that any change in pressure at any point within a confined fluid will be transmitted without loss to all other points of the fluid.

Static pressure in a fluid is referred to as **hydrostatic pressure**, where $p = h \rho g$ (pascals).

Absolute pressure = gauge pressure + atmospheric pressure.

Hydrostatic pressure arising from gravity influences blood pressure in different parts of the body and the effect is particularly noticeable in different body positions such as lying, sitting and standing.

If a body is wholly or partially immersed in a liquid, it experiences a vertical **buoyancy force** equal and opposite to the weight of liquid that would occupy the space enclosed by the immersed part of the body (weight of the displaced liquid), and this up-thrust acts through the **centre of buoyancy**, which is the centre of gravity of the displaced liquid. This is known as **Archimedes' principle**.

The apparent weight of a body in water is less than that in air because of the up-thrust of the buoyancy force.

Weight always acts vertically downwards and buoyancy force always acts vertically upwards. Consequently, moments of force arising from buoyancy forces acting on limbs that are submerged in water act contrary to moments which arise from the weight of the limb.

Fluid motion in which one fluid layer or lamina slides smoothly over another without turbulence is called **laminar** or **streamlined flow**.

Newton's **law of viscosity** relates shear stress and viscosity to the rate of angular deformation of the fluid, which is described in terms of the rate of change of velocity of the fluid normal to the velocity, i.e.

$$\tau = \eta \frac{\Delta v}{\Delta y} \text{ (Pa)}$$

where

τ = shear stress
η = viscosity (kg m^{-1} s^{-1}) and
$\dfrac{\Delta v}{\Delta y}$ = rate of change in velocity of the fluid normal to the velocity.

Turbulence occurs when fluid swirls and mixes, causing dissipation of mechanical energy, and is related to an increase in fluid velocity past a critical threshold value. An expression known as **Reynold's number** (R) is used to estimate whether flow will be laminar or turbulent.

The variables which determine the resistance to flow of an incompressible fluid in a tube when the flow is laminar, i.e. streamlined, are related in **Poiseuille's law**. This equation illustrates the dominant effect of the radius of the tube in controlling resistance to flow and is helpful in explaining the effect of vasoconstriction and vasodilation in the vascular system.

8.10   TUTORIAL PROBLEMS

1. The following factors affect the pressure at the bottom of an open water container; true or false?
    (a) volume of water;
    (b) total weight of water;
    (c) weight density of water;
    (d) depth of water;
    (e) shape of container.

2. (a) A 5 kg block rests on a 10 kg block which rests on the base of an empty water tank. Find the force exerted:
        (i)   by the 5 kg block on the 10 kg block;
        (ii) by the 10 kg block on the 5 kg block;
        (iii) by the 10 kg block on the base of the tank;
        (iv) by the base of the tank on the 10 kg block.

    Briefly state beside each answer the premise(s) on which the answer is based.

    (b) The blocks referred to in (a) above are now completely covered by a liquid whose density is half that of the blocks. Find the force exerted:
        (i)   by the 5 kg block on the 10 kg block;
        (ii) by the 10 kg block on the 5 kg block;
        (iii) by the 10 kg block on the base of the tank;
        (iv) by the base of the tank on the 10 kg block.

    (c) With reference to the problem stated in (b) what minimum vertical force would be required to just raise the 5 kg block clear of the 10 kg block?

3. (a) During hydrotherapy a patient slowly moves a fully extended limb upwards from a vertical position to a horizontal position while still maintaining it under the surface of the water; are the following statements true or false? (Assume that the density of the limb is greater than that of the water.)
        (i)   The patient would require to exert more effort than that required to perform the same exercise out of water.
        (ii) The force of buoyancy would increase as the limb approached the horizontal.
        (iii) If the limb is in effect streamlined the frictional resistance of the water will be independent of the velocity of movement.

    (b) Briefly state the premise(s) for each of your answers in (a).

4. 'It is usually inadvisable to put patients with a vital lung capacity of less than 1500 cm^3 into a pool.'
    'Swelling will be reduced more easily if exercises are given well below the surface of the water.'

    Briefly explain, in your own words, what hydrostatic principle(s) underlie the above statements.

5. A body is suspended from a spring balance and registers a weight of 6 N. When the body is completely immersed in water the reading of the balance shows 4 N. Find the relative density of the body.

6. A body of weight 12 N is suspended from a spring balance. The reading of the balance is 10 N when the body is totally immersed in water and 10.5 N when the body is totally immersed in another liquid. Find the relative density of the body and the unknown liquid.

Appendix: where next?

There is no simple single solution to acquiring the level of knowledge of biomechanics most appropriate to the individual reader. Different needs, backgrounds and abilities have to be addressed by referring to both breadth and depth of the material available.

Mechanics is traditionally viewed as a part of physics, primarily because the mathematics used in developing the various branches of physics is similar, involving, at an elementary level, geometry, algebra and trigonometry and, at a more advanced level, calculus and methods for handling three-dimensional vectors and related data. For an insight into the scope of medical physics problems extending beyond biomechanics, physical scientists and engineers entering the healthcare field may find some of the physics texts aimed at health care students[1,2,3] useful in providing a healthcare context to topics already dealt with at secondary school or first-year University level.

While physical scientists and engineers have the advantage of a sound background in mathematics, which is often necessary to understand the details of primary sources of information in journals such as the *Journal of Biomechanics*, they have the disadvantage in most cases of a lack of even basic terminology in anatomy and physiology; texts such as Palastanga *et al*.[4] and Basmajian[5] could be useful for these readers.

Healthcare students will in many cases be introduced to biomechanics as a part of the broader discipline of kinesiology and a number of kinesiology text books include material on mechanical and biomechanical principles.[6,7] A knowledge of trigonometry would be an advantage for any reader using the classical text by Williams and Lissner, which has been extended and updated by Le Veau.[8]

Access to a good library is essential for the study of any subject and I would strongly advise all readers to take advantage of the range of resources that are now available in all good libraries. The book by Payton[9] on research methods has a very informative chapter on 'the library as a tool', which, fortuitously, uses biomechanics as the search topic example. In addition to printed material there is also a growing resource of audio-visual and multimedia material available on topics such as gait analysis; information is generally provided in publishers' catalogues and these should be available in libraries or bookstores.

A problem facing both students and practising professionals today is that as more information becomes available and as information technology provides access to sources of data more rapidly, the problems of selection and interpretation of relevant, valid and reliable information increase.

Databases on CD-ROM are very extensive; the index alone to CD-ROM databases (which are referred to as off-line) is a 500 page A4 volume. The equivalent index for on-line databases (i.e. databases connected to some remote central computer) is about 400 pages.

Examples of particularly relevant computer based databases include the following.

- **Medline**, the CD-ROM version of *Index Medicus*, covering material from over 4000 medical or medically-related journals.
- **Bookbank**, the CD-ROM version of books in print, containing references to over 640 000 books published in the UK and Western Europe.
- There are three databases on, respectively, **Occupational Therapy**, **Physiotherapy** and **Rehabilitation**. These are PC-based databases produced from the specialist occupational therapy, physiotherapy and rehabilitation journals held in the British Library.
- **RECAL Database**, also a PC-based database, produced from the specialist journals held in the National Centre for Training and Education in Prosthetics and Orthotics at the University of Strathclyde, Glasgow.
- **Focus on Sports Science and Medicine** from ISI (Institute for Scientific Information, USA).

Browsing over printed source material on databases, textbooks in specific topic areas and specialized journals is still well worthwhile despite the attraction of computer technology. There are books on biomechanics related to particular topics or specialities such as gait analysis,[10] orthopaedics,[11-13] the cardiovascular system,[14] the respiratory system,[15] exercise,[16] sports[17,18] and so forth. Of course, browsing can also be undertaken via computer too and systems such as OPAC (On-line Public Access Catalogue), which will also allow access to other library OPACs and the Internet will enable users to print out lists of possible books and journals of interest and lead the searcher to the correct library shelves for further browsing.

Professional bodies or local universities or colleges should be able to advise on the existence of special interest groups who may be able to provide specific advice on relevant sources of information or on part-time and distance-learning courses in biomechanics. Special interest groups now use e-mail (electronic mail via computer) to exchange information. Some very innovative multimedia material on biomechanics, which uses text, images, audio and animation, is being developed at a number of centres, including the four universities in the Glasgow area in Scotland, for use on local computer based networks.

At national and international level there are the American Society of Biomechanics, the European Society of Biomechanics and the International Society of Biomechanics. In the UK the Biological Engineering Society (now part of the Institute of Physics and Engineering in Medicine) has provided a valuable focus for biomechanics within the broader area of bioengineering.

In addition to journals such as Clinical Biomechanics and the Journal of Biomechanics, journals dealing with bioengineering, exercise, orthopaedics, occupational therapy, orthotics and prosthetics, physiotherapy, podiatry, rehabilitation and sports often include articles and review articles on biomechanics. Most of these journals also provide information on forthcoming conferences and meetings in the form of a calendar of events. There is a wealth of material on biomechanics and it is a fascinating discipline to pursue and develop.

Good luck!

REFERENCES

1. Burns DM and MacDonald SGG. *Physics for Biology and Pre-Medical Students*. New York: Addison-Wesley, 1975.
2. Nave CR and Nave BC. *Physics for the Health Sciences*. Philadelphia: WB Saunders, 1985.
3. Urone PP. *Physics with Health Science Applications*. New York: Harper & Row, 1986.
4. Palastanga N, Field A and Soames R. *Anatomy and Human Movement. Structure and Functions*. London: Butterworth-Heinemann, 1991.
5. Basmajian JV. *Muscles Alive*. Baltimore: Williams & Wilkins, 1985.
6. Luttgens K and Wells KF. *Kinesiology: Scientific Basis of Human Motion*. Philadelphia: WB Saunders, 1982.
7. Enoka RM. *Neuromechanical Basis of Kinesiology*. Human Kinetics, 1994.
8. Le Veau B. *Williams and Lissner's Biomechanics of Human Motion*. Philadelphia: WB Saunders, 1992.
9. Payton OD. *Research. The Validation of Clinical Practice*. Philadelphia: FA Davis, 1994.
10. Whittle M. *Gait Analysis: An Introduction*. London: Butterworth-Heinemann, 1991.
11. Cochran GA. *A Primer of Orthopaedic Biomechanics*. Edinburgh: Churchill Livingstone, 1982.
12. Nordin M and Frankel VH. *Basic Biomechanics of the Skeletal System*. Philadelphia: Lea & Febiger, 1989.
13. Wright V and Radin E. *Mechanics of Human Joints: Physiology, Pathophysiology and Treatment*. Cleveland, OH: Marcel Dekker, 1993.
14. Chandran KB. *Cardiovascular Biomechanics*. New York: New York, 1992.
15. Epstein MA and Ligas JR (eds). *Respiratory Biomechanics: Engineering Analysis of Structure and Function*. New York: Springer-Verlag, 1990.
16. Johnson AT. *Biomechanics and Exercise Physiology*. New York: John Wiley, 1991.
17. Watkins J. *An Introduction to the Mechanics of Human Movement*. Lancaster: MTP Press, 1990.
18. Vaughan CL. *Biomechanics and Sport*. Boca Raton, FL: CRC Press, 1989.

Answers to tutorial problems

CHAPTER 1

2. (a) Of the order of three times body weight, i.e. 1500 N.
   (b) Leverage or moment of force.
   (c) Lean his/her trunk toward the supporting hip to minimize leverage.
3. (a) Description of the motion of a body without reference to the forces causing motion.
   (b) Gait analysis.
4. A force associated with acceleration or deceleration of a body, for example during impact.

CHAPTER 2

1. See Figure A.1.
   The correct SI unit for weight is the newton (Note that lower case is used for the initial letter for all units named after people although upper case is used for the symbols, e.g. N).

2.

Quantity	SI unit	Unit symbol
Length	metre	m
Mass	kilogram	kg
Time	second	s
Force	newton	N
Weight	newton	N

3. The difficulty arises in **accelerating** the object from rest. The force required to accelerate the object is directly proportional to its mass ($F = m\,a$) and as weight is also directly proportional to mass ($W = m\,g$); a 'heavy' object is defined as having a greater mass. Once the object is moving at a desired velocity no net force is required to maintain motion.
4. (a) 700 N
   (b) 40 N
   (c) 5 N
   (d) 1 N

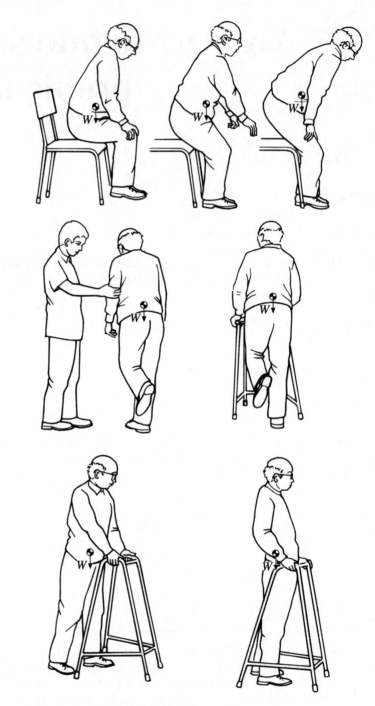

Figure A.1 Answer to tutorial problem 1.

(e) 3.56×10^{-3} N

1 kg = 1000 g

5. The four characteristics needed to fully describe a force are magnitude, line of action, direction (or sense) and point of application.
6. They are balanced. The forces are cancelling each other out, i.e. there is no net force acting.
7. Both magnitude and direction must be specified to describe a vector quantity such as force.
8. These terms describe the equal and opposite forces acting between two interacting bodies.
9. Moment of force is the turning effect of a force.
10. Caution is required because the internal muscle and joint reaction forces in each case may be different as a result of internal leverage within the bodies.

CHAPTER 3

1. (a) See Figure A.2.
   (b) When seated (Figure A.2(i, left), the chair legs form part of the base of support. The patient is extrinsically stable. As the patient egresses from the chair (Figure A.2(i, centre) his base of support is reduced to his feet only. To be extrinsically stable his line of gravity must lie within this base. If the line of gravity lies behind his heels he will tend to fall back into the chair. Because this patient cannot extend his trunk in relation to his thighs (weak hip extensors), he tries to use momentum to raise his upper body by swinging his arms forward. If, as a result, his line of gravity passes in front of his toes he will tend to fall forward. Figure A.2 (right): As the line of gravity lies within the base of support the patient is extrinsically stable. However, because of weak hip extensors he can only extend his trunk by using his arms as struts; he is intrinsically unstable. When his arms are straight (full extension at the elbows) he has reached the limit of trunk extension. A chair with high arm rests would allow him to push up into standing position.

   Figure A.2(ii): When standing on both feet the line of gravity passes through the centre of the base of support. As the patient raises his left leg off the floor his body weight will tend to cause him to fall over to the left. Normally, the muscles passing over the right hip (the abductors) will contract, pulling the trunk over to the right side. Extrinsic stability will be achieved if the line of gravity moves to the right, passing through the reduced base of support, i.e. his right foot. As this patient has weak hip abductors he is intrinsically and extrinsically unstable when standing on one leg. He requires external support in the form of an aide or an aid.

   Figure A.2(iii): The walking frame increases the patient's base of support and hence extrinsic stability when it is in contact with the floor. This aid nevertheless has to be lifted to move forward. Walking,

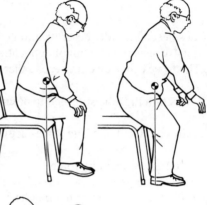

(i)

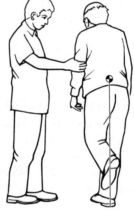
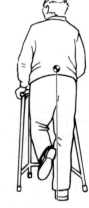

(ii)

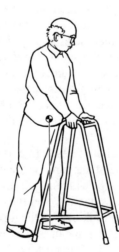
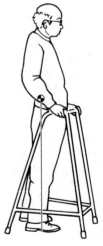

(iii)

Figure A.2 Answer to tutorial problem 1.

with or without an aid, involves a 'controlled loss of balance' and can not be analysed solely in terms of static equilibrium.

2. See Figure A.3.

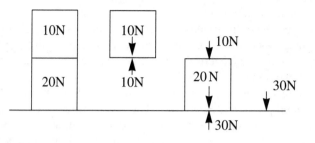

Figure A.3 Answer to tutorial problem 2.

3. (a) The required force, i.e. the effort, increases.
   (b) The principle of moments of force. As the moment arm (L) decreases, i.e. the leverage decreases, the required force (F) must increase to produce the same moment of force ($M = F \times L$) to overcome the resistance to motion of the door.
4. (a) The body tends to fall forward.
   (b) As the trunk bends forward, the centre of gravity of the body moves forward. The subject would normally counter this by moving the buttocks backwards so that the line of gravity continues to pass through the base of support, but the wall prevents this. The line of gravity passes in front of the toes outside the base of support; the body is now extrinsically unstable.
5. (a) See Figure A.4.
   (b) Clockwise.
   (c) By a counter-clockwise moment produced by the hip extensor muscles.

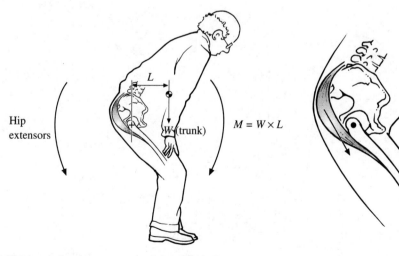

Figure A.4 Answer to tutorial problem 5.

CHAPTER 4

1. (a) Ground reaction force is a force equal and opposite to the action force being applied to the ground by the foot. Newton's third law provides a statement on action–reaction forces.

   (b) A force can be illustrated precisely by a vector whose length represents the magnitude of the force and whose direction (i.e. line of action and sense) represents that of the force, as illustrated in Figure A.5.

   (c) As illustrated in Figure A.5.

2. This is a very basic biomechanical 'model' which raises a number of fundamental problems. How do we know what forces are acting and what their characteristics are (i.e. magnitude, line of action, direction, point of application)? With reference to Figure A.6 (a), weight (W) always acts vertically downwards through the centre of gravity of the object. Even without access to research data on the location of the centre of gravity of body segments a reasonable guess would place it about one third of the way along the length of the forearm. Muscles can only pull, thus, the force generated by the muscle must act upwards and the point of application is the point of attachment of the tendon to the bones in the forearm. This can be estimated by examining anatomical models and reference texts but it is obviously closer to the axis of rotation of the

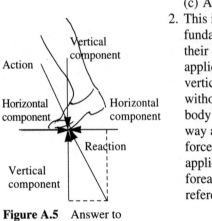

Figure A.5 Answer to tutorial problem 1(b).

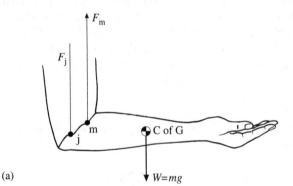

(a)

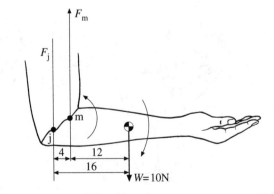

(b)

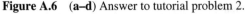

Figure A.6 (**a–d**) Answer to tutorial problem 2.

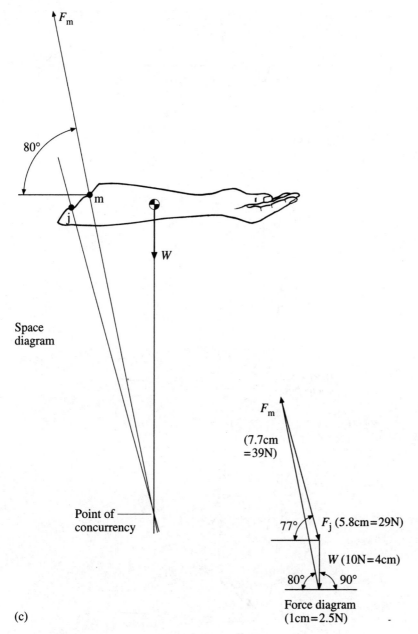

(c)

Figure A.6 continued

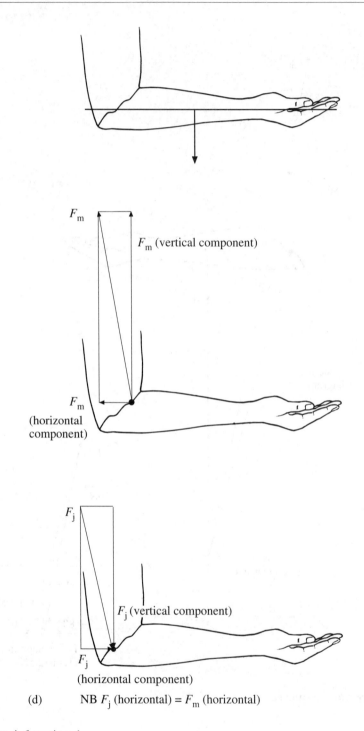

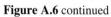

(d)   NB F_j (horizontal) = F_m (horizontal)

Figure A.6 continued

elbow joint than the centre of gravity of the arm is (measurement of the electrical activity which accompanies muscle contraction can be used to determine which muscles are contracting in given situations). In some situations, if other significant forces exist because more than one muscle is acting or because of the stretching of ligaments around a joint, the problem may not be amenable to simple static analysis. The location of the 'point' of application of the force within the elbow joint is again an estimate. The elbow joint, although described as a 'hinge type' joint, has quite complex articulating surfaces; the contact force will be distributed over an area of the articulating surfaces. Its downward direction can, however, be confirmed by calculations as follows.

(a) With reference to Figure A.6 (b), three forces are assumed to be acting.

$$W = m \times g$$
$$= 1 \times 10$$
$$= 10 \text{ N}$$

The point of application, line of action, and direction of F_m is known but not its magnitude.

At this stage only the 'point' of application and line of action F_j are known; as W and F_m are vertical, F_j must also be vertical otherwise it would provide an unbalanced horizontal force, i.e. ΣF horizontal = 0. For static equilibrium ΣF vertical = 0 and $\Sigma M = 0$.

By taking moments about a point, through which the line of action of one of the unknown forces passes, this unknown is eliminated from the equation. Thus, by taking moments about point j, F_m can be determined; clockwise moments are taken as positive.

$$-(F_m \times 4) + (W \times 16) = 0$$
$$-(F_m \times 4) + (10 \times 16) = 0$$

$$F_m = \frac{10 \times 16}{4}$$

$$F_m = 40 \text{N}$$

(b) With reference to Figure A.6(c) the numerical solution to the problem can be determined by using both the concept of concurrency of three non-parallel forces and by constructing a polygon of forces. An accurate space diagram (with a scale of say 1:2) is required to find the point of concurrency. The lines of action of W and F_m are extended and a line drawn from the point of concurrency to the point of application of F_j

A force diagram is then constructed using the force polygon method of vector additon (using a scale of say 1 cm = 2.5 N). The line of action of all three forces are now known and the magnitude of W (10 N). W is first drawn to scale and the lines of action of F_m and F_j added to W to provide a triangle by placing the tail of F_m at the head W and the tail of F_j at the head of F_m. For the body to be in equilibrium the polygon (which is a triangle in this case) must close.

By measurement: F_m = 39 N (acting at 80 degrees to the horizontal in an upward direction, as given); F_j = 28 N acting at 77 degrees to the horizontal in a downward direction, as shown.

The small angles between the force vectors in this example can lead to inaccuracies in measurement, and calculations using trigonometry would eliminate such errors. Nevertheless the final results must reflect the accuracy of the initial data and assumptions.

Figure A.6 (d) summaries the vertical and horizontal components of the forces W, F_m and F_j. W has no horizontal component, thus the horizontal forces arising from F_m and F_j are equal and opposite.

3. With reference to Figure A.7, if the limb is supported at a point then movement involves displacing the cords supporting the limb through an angle, say θ; this induces a horizontal component of force, H, which will tend to pull the limb back into its original position; the freely swinging support reduces the resistance to movement during the movement and allows the cord to remain vertical after movement.

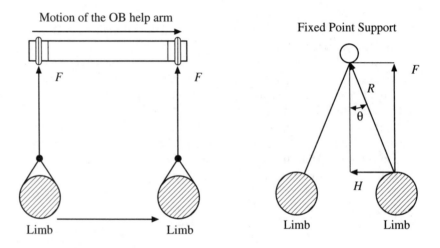

Figure A.7   Answer to tutorial problem 4.

4. Patients who suffer pain at the patellofemoral joint often complain that the pain is most intense when (a) walking down stairs; and (b) rising from a chair (See Figure A.8). In both activities the knee is in a flexed position when weight is being borne by the lower limbs and the line of gravity of the patient's body weight passes behind the knee joints. This tends to flex the knees. Contraction of the muscles, the knee extensors, which resist this 'buckling' action, also pull the patella tighter against the femur, increasing the pressure on the patellofemoral joint. The more the knee is flexed during weight bearing the greater the resultant force acting on the patellofemoral joint; a parallelogram of forces illustrates this effect quite clearly. People seldom lean forward when descending stairs for fear of falling. When ascending stairs, leaning forward may assist in placing the line of gravity in front of the knee joint, reducing pressure on the patellofemoral joint.

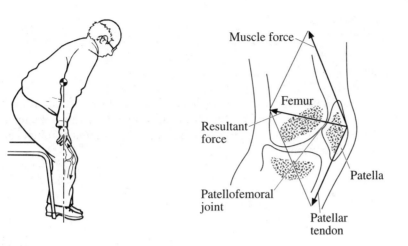

Figure A.8   Answer to tutorial problem 4.

CHAPTER 5

1. The increased leverage means that a smaller force can be applied to provide the same turning effect, i.e. the same moment of force ($M = F \times L$).

2. (a) Work done = Force $\times$ displacement of force
   $$= m \times g \times \text{height}$$
   $$= 2 \text{ (kg)} \times 10\text{(m s}^{-2}) \times 1\text{(m)}$$
   $$= 20 \text{ Nm (or J)}$$

   (b) Average power = $\dfrac{\text{work done}}{\text{time taken}}$
   $$= \frac{20 \text{ (J)}}{0.5 \text{ (s)}}$$
   $$= 40 \text{ W}$$

3. With reference to Figure A.12:
   $f = \mu \times N$
   $N = F_y$
   f must be greater than F_x if slipping is to be avoided, thus
   $F_x \leqslant \mu \times F_y$
   where μ is the coefficient of static friction.

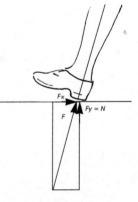

Figure A.12   Answer to tutorial problem 3.

4. With reference to Figure A.13:
   $W = m g$
   $$= 80 \times 10$$
   $$= 800 \text{ N.}$$
   The therapist must apply a force E, equal and opposite to the component of W that is acting down the incline F. Also by proportion:
   $\dfrac{F}{W} = \dfrac{1}{5}$
   $F = \dfrac{W}{5}$

$$F = \frac{800}{5}$$

$F = 160 \text{ N}$

and as $E = - F$

$\therefore E = 160 \text{ N}$ acting up the incline.

Friction always opposes motion. When E is less than F, friction assists the therapist in preventing the wheelchair from rolling down the incline. As E exceeds F, friction increases the effort (E) required to initiate and maintain motion.

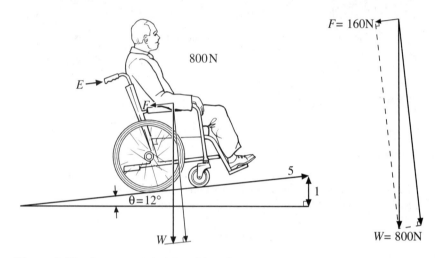

Figure A.13 Answer to tutorial problem 4.

5. With reference to Figure A.14, when the plane is horizontal the effort, E, required for motion of the limb is equal to that required to overcome friction and inertia of the limb. As the plane is inclined these forces are still required but additional force, E (effort), is required to overcome the component, W_p, of the weight of the limb, W, which is tending to accelerate the limb down the plane.

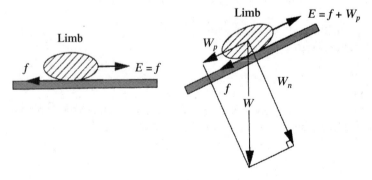
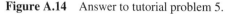

Figure A.14 Answer to tutorial problem 5.

6. System 1 requires most effort, a force equal to W to be applied, whereas System 2 which incorporates a moveable pulley requires a force equal to $W/2$ (Figure A.15).

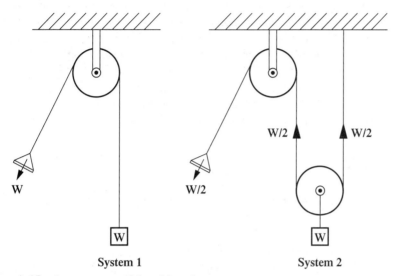

| System 1 | System 2 |

Figure A.15 Answer to tutorial problem 6.

7. (a) 20 kg.
   (b) 40 kg.

CHAPTER 6

1. Load refers to the amount of force acting on one side of a section of a body. Stress refers to the load per unit area acting on a plane within a body.
2. Stress relates to load and strain to deformation.
3. (a) Tangent modulus of elasticity is used to determine the stiffness of a material at a point which only approximates linearity.
   (b) Because of the limited linear response of human tissue to load.
4. Being more compliant than the outer shell of compact bone, cancellous bone may attenuate impulsive forces and protect the joints.
5. The orientation of collagen along the axis of the structure provides resistance to tensile loads but limited resistance to bending or shearing loads.
6. Stretching of the outer surface or 'membrane' of a body adjacent to an area of compression will cause tensile stress.
7. Fluid flow delays the deformation, enhancing the time-dependent viscoelastic response of the load bearing surface in joints.
8. Damage to the ligament occurs at this point. If it is necessary to permanently lengthen a ligamentous structure this can only be achieved by stretching it beyond the yield point.

9. Greater deformation of connective tissue is achieved at a low strain rate; being viscoelastic it is strain-rate-dependent.

10. Bending and torsion of structures result in non-uniform stresses across sections of the structure that vary from zero at some axis within the section to maxima at the outer surfaces. The influence of the geometrical properties of cross-sections of structures are included in a factor called the area moment of inertia in bending and the polar moment of inertia in torsion.

11. Hardness is a measure of resistance to indentation or scoring of the surface and defects such as scratches on the surface can impair the bearing surface and lead to stress concentrations.

CHAPTER 7

1. (a) Work done = force × distance
$$= 6 \times 10 \times 0.3$$
$$= 18 \text{ J}$$

(b) Average power = $\dfrac{\text{work done}}{\text{time taken}}$
$$= \dfrac{18}{2}$$
$$= 9 \text{ W}$$

2. Work done = average force × displacement
$$= \dfrac{40}{2} \times 0.5$$
$$= 10 \text{ J}$$

3. (a) Average velocity, $\omega = \dfrac{0.2(\text{rad})}{0.2(\text{s})}$
$$\omega = 1 \text{ rad s}^{-1}$$
$$\omega_f = 2 \omega$$
$$= 2 \text{ rad s}^{-1}$$

Therefore the value of the angular velocity of the limb after 0.2 s is 2 rad s⁻¹.

(b)
$$\alpha = \dfrac{\omega_f - \omega_i}{t}$$
$$= \dfrac{2 - 0}{0.2}$$
$$= 10 \text{ rad s}^{-2}.$$

Therefore the value of the constant angular acceleration of the limb during this part of the swing is 10 rad s⁻².

4. During circular motion at constant angular velocity the object will be subject to centripetal acceleration.

5. The compliant nature of the surface underfoot extends the length of time (Δt) required to generate sufficient ground reaction force (F) necessary for both the 'push off' and 'heel-strike' actions involved in walking. This can be expressed in terms of Newton's second law in its 'impulse equation' form:

$$F = \frac{m \times \Delta v}{\Delta t}$$

Part of the energy expended in compressing the compliant surface is dissipated in the form of heat.

6. Pushing the wheelchair on a flat surface at a constant velocity will only require sufficient force to overcome rolling friction. Starting, stopping and changing direction will all require forces to be applied by the attendant proportional to the mass of patient and wheelchair and these will be exacerbated on inclined surfaces.

7. (a) Impact force increases directly as mass increases.
   (b) Impact force increases as the velocity and hence momentum just prior to impact increases; the velocity in turn is directly proportional to the square root of height of fall.
   (c) The average force during impact increases as the time interval to bring the body to rest decreases; the force consequently increases as the compliance decreases.

8. Inertia is a measure of the resistance that a body offers to acceleration which depends upon the mass of the body. Moment of inertia is a measure of the resistance that a body offers to angular acceleration; it depends upon the mass of the body and the distribution of the mass with respect to the body's axis of rotation.

CHAPTER 8

1. (a) False
   (b) False
   (c) True
   (d) True
   (e) False.
2. (a) (i) $W = m\,g = 5 \times 10 = 50$ N vertically downward (equilibrium and Newton's second and third laws)
   (ii) 50 N vertically upward (equilibrium and Newton's third law)
   (iii) $(10 \times 10) + 50$
       $= 100 + 50 = 150$ N vertically downward (equilibrium and Newton's second and third laws)
   (iv) 150 N vertically upward (equilibrium and Newton's third law).
   (b) (i) Weight (50 N) $-$ buoyancy force (25 N) $= 25$ N downwards.
   (ii) 25 N (Newton's third law)
   (iii) 125 N $-$ 50 N $= 75$ N
   (iv) 75 N (Newton's third law).
   (c) 25 N provided the block remains immersed in the liquid.
3. (a) (i) False
   (ii) False
   (iii) False.
   (b) (i) Force of buoyancy would assist limb.
   (ii) Force of buoyancy is independent of depth under water once fully submerged.

(iii) Streamlined flow resistance depends on velocity.

4. • Hydrostatic pressure increases with depth.
   • Pressure in a liquid is transmitted equally in all directions at a given point.
   • Hydrostatic pressure acts normal to the surface of immersed object. Thus hydrostatic pressure would tend to resist expansion of chest; would tend to decrease swelling.

5. The buoyancy force (up-thrust) is (6 N − 4 N) = 2 N and the relative density of the body is:

   weight of body/ buoyancy force, i.e. 6 N /2 N = 3.

6. The up-thrust on the body in water is 12 − 10 = 2 N, and this gives the weight of an equal volume of water. Therefore:

   relative density of the body = $\dfrac{12 \text{ N}}{2 \text{ N}}$ = 6.

   The up-thrust when the body is immersed in the liquid is 1.5 N. This means that the volume occupied by the body has a weight of 2 N for water and 1.5 N for the liquid. Therefore the relative density of the liquid is 1.5 N/2 N = 0.75. (The density of the body is 6000 kg/cubic metre and the density of the liquid is 750 kg/cubic metre.)

LLYFRGELL COLEG MENAI LIBRARY
SAFLE FFRIDDOEDD SITE
BANGOR GWYNEDD LL57 2TP

Index